Case Studies In Interventional Cardiology

CASE STUDIES IN INTERVENTIONAL CARDIOLOGY

Edited by

Martin T Rothman FRCP FESC FACC
Professor of Interventional Cardiology
Consultant Cardiologist
London Chest Hospital
London
UK

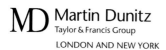
Martin Dunitz
Taylor & Francis Group
LONDON AND NEW YORK

© 2004 Martin Dunitz, an imprint of Taylor & Francis Group

First published in the United Kingdom in 2004
by Martin Dunitz, an imprint of Taylor and Francis Group, 11 New Fetter Lane,
London EC4P 4EE

Tel.:	+44 (0) 20 7583 9855
Fax.:	+44 (0) 20 7842 2298
E-mail:	info@dunitz.co.uk
Website:	http://www.dunitz.co.uk

A CIP record for this book is available from the British Library.

ISBN 1 84184 020 3

Distributed in the USA by
Fulfilment Center
Taylor & Francis
10650 Toebben Drive
Independence, KY 41051, USA
Toll Free Tel.: +1 800 634 7064
E-mail: taylorandfrancis@thomsonlearning.com

Distributed in Canada by
Taylor & Francis
74 Rolark Drive
Scarborough, Ontario M1R 4G2, Canada
Toll Free Tel.: +1 877 226 2237
E-mail: tal_fran@istar.ca

Distributed in the rest of the world by
Thomson Publishing Services
Cheriton House
North Way
Andover, Hampshire SP10 5BE, UK
Tel.:   +44 (0)1264 332424
E-mail: salesorder.tandf@thomsonpublishingservices.co.uk

Composition by 𝍐 Tek-Art

Printed and bound in Great Britain by the Cromwell Press, Trowbridge

Contents

v

CONTRIBUTORS

Rajpal K Abhaichand MD DM FICPS
Consultant Interventional Cardiologist
Fellow, Institut Cardiovasculaire Paris Sud
Paris
FRANCE

Alexandre Abizaid MD PhD
Director, Intravascular Ultrasound Core Lab
Institute Dante Pazzanese of Cardiology
Sao Paulo
BRAZIL

Andrea S Abizaid MD PhD
Co-Director, Intravascular Ultrasound Core Lab
Institute Dante Pazzanese of Cardiology
Sao Paulo
BRAZIL

David Antoniucci MD
Head, Division of Cardiology
Careggi Hospital
Florence
ITALY

Antonio L Bartorelli MD
Associate Professor of Cardiology and
Director, Catheterization Laboratory
Institute of Cardiology
University of Milan
Centro Cardiologico Monzino IRCCS
Milan
ITALY

Andreas Baumbach
Department of Cardiology
Bristol Royal Infirmary
Bristol
UK

Dietrich Baumgart MD
Division of Cardiology
Centre of Internal Medicine
University of Essen
Hufelandstr 55
D-45122 Essen
GERMANY

Raphael Beyar MD
Division of Invasive Cardiology
Rambam Medical Center
and Technion – Israel Institute of Technology
Haifa
ISRAEL

Clemens von Birgelen MD PhD
Consultant Cardiologist
and Director of Invasive Ultrasound Program
Department of Cardiology
Hôpital de la Tour
Geneva
SWITZERLAND

Antoine Bloch MD
Director, Non-invasive Cardiology
Department of Cardiology
Hôpital de la Tour
Geneva
SWITZERLAND

Bruce R Brodie MD
Clinical Professor of Medicine
University of North Carolina Teaching
Service
Moses Cone Hospital
Director, Le Bauer Cardiovascular Research
Foundation
Greensboro, NC
USA

Bernard de Bruyne MD PhD
Cardiovascular Center Aalst
Moorselbaan 164
B-9300 Aalst
Belgium

Prof. Dr Thomas Budde
Clinic for Internal Medicine 1
Alfried-Krupp-Krankenhaus
45117 Essen
GERMANY

Edoardo Camenzind MD
Director of Interventional Cardiology
Cardiology Department
University Hospital
Geneva
SWITZERLAND

Manoel Cano MD
Staff, Interventional Cardiology
Institute Dante Pazzanese of Cardiology
Sao Paulo
BRAZIL

Qi-Ling Cao
Senior Research Scientist
University of Chicago
Chicago, IL
USA

Stephane G Carlier MD PhD
Thoraxcenter
Erasmus Medical Center
Rotterdam
THE NETHERLANDS

M Centemero MD
Staff, Clinical Cardiology
Institute Dante Pazzanese of Cardiology
Sao Paulo
BRAZIL

A Chaves MD
Staff, Clinical Cardiology
Institute Dante Pazzanese of Cardiology
Sao Paulo
BRAZIL

Antonio Colombo MD
Director, Cardiac Catheterization Laboratory
EMO Centro Cuore Columbus
Milan
ITALY

Marco A Costa MD
Division of Cardiology
University of Florida, Shands Jacksonville
655 W 8th St
Jacksonville FL 32209
USA

Nicholas Curzen BM (Hons) PhD MRCP FESC
Consultant Cardiologist
Manchester Heart Centre
Manchester Royal Infirmary
Manchester
UK

George Dangas MD PhD
Director, Academic Affairs and Investigational
Pharmacology
Cardiovascular Research Foundation
New York, NY
USA

Rainer Dietz
Franz Volhard Clinic
Wiltberg Strasse 50
13125 Berlin
GERMANY

Olaf Dirsch
Department of Cardiology
Essen University
Essen
GERMANY

Dr Holger Eggebrecht
Cardiology Clinic
University Essen
45122 Essen
GERMANY

Stephen Ellis
Director, Sones Cardiac Catheterization
Laboratories
Department of Cardiology
Cleveland Clinic Foundation
Cleveland, OH
USA

Raimund Erbel MD
Professor of Internal Medicine
Consultant Cardiologist and
Director, Division of Cardiology
Essen University
Department of Cardiology
Essen
GERMANY

Andrew Farb MD
Staff Cardiovascular Pathologist
Department of Cardiovascular Pathology
Armed Forces Institute of Pathology
Washington DC
USA

Fausto Feres MD PhD
Staff, Interventional Cardiology
Institute Dante Pazzanese of Cardiology
Sao Paulo
BRAZIL

Pim de Feijter MD
Professor, Thoraxcenter, Erasmus Medical
Center, Rotterdam
PO Box 2040
3000 CA Rotterdam
THE NETHERLANDS

Tim A Fischell
Borgess Research Institute
1521 Gull Road
Kalamazoo, MI 49048
USA

Malcolm T Foster
Borgess Research Institute
1521 Gull Road
Kalamazoo, MI 49048
USA

Anthony H Gershlick
Consultant Cardiologist
Department of Cardiology
Glenfield Hospital
Leicester
UK

Wim J van der Giessen MD PhD
Department of Coronary Diagnostics and
Intervention
Thoraxcenter
University Hospital Dijkzigt
Rotterdam
THE NETHERLANDS

Mario Gössl MD
Resident in Cardiology
Essen University
Department of Cardiology
Essen
GERMANY

C Michael Gross MD
Head, Department of Interventional
Cardiology and Angiology
HELIOS Clinic Berlin, Franz-Volhard-Clinic
Charité Berlin, Campus Buch
D-13125 Berlin
GERMANY

Michael Haude MD
Cardiology Clinic
University of Essen
45122 Essen
GERMANY

Niall A Herity
Royal Victoria Hospital
Grosvenor Road
BELFAST BT12 6BA

Joerg Herrmann MD
Cardiology Clinic
University Essen
45122 Essen
Germany

Ziyad M Hijazi MD MPH FAAP FACC FSCAI FESC
Chief, Section of Pediatric Cardiology
Professor of Pediatrics and Medicine
The University of Chicago
Chicago, IL
USA

John McB Hodgson MD FACC FSCAI
Director, Invasive Cardiology
Heart and Vascular Center
MetroHealth Medical Center
Cleveland, OH
USA

Rainer Hoffmann MD FESC
Director of Interventional Cardiology
Medical Clinic 1
University of Aachen
Aachen
GERMANY

Thomas A Ischinger MD FACC FESC
Professor of Medicine/Cardiology
Klinikum Bogenhausen
Division of Cardiology
81925 Munich
GERMANY

Karl S Karsch MD
Department of Cardiology
Bristol Royal Infirmary
Bristol
UK

I Patrick Kay MBChB PhD FRACP FESC
Interventional Cardiologist
Cardiology Department
Dunedin Hospital
GT King St
Dunedin
NEW ZEALAND

Morton J Kern MD
Professor of Medicine
St Louis University
Director, JG Mudd Cardiac Catheterization
Laboratory
St Louis, MO
USA

Yoshio Kobayashi MD
Director, Intravascular Ultrasound Laboratory
Cardiovascular Research Foundation
Lenox Hill Heart and Vascular Institute
New York, NY
USA

Chris L de Korte PhD
Experimental Echocardiography
Erasmus Medical Center
Rotterdam
THE NETHERLANDS

Jochen Krämer MD
Attendant, Department of Interventional
Cardiology and Angiology
HELIOS Clinic Berlin, Franz-Volhard-Clinic
Charité Berlin, Campus Buch
D-13125 Berlin
GERMANY

Michael JB Kutryk MD PhD FRCPC
Assistant Professor
Division of Cardiology
St Michael's Hospital
Toronto, ONT
CANADA

Glenn van Langenhove MD
Department of Interventional Cardiology
Thoraxcenter Rotterdam
Academic Hospital Dijkzigt
Erasmus University
THE NETHERLANDS

Michael Lauer MD
Borgess Research Institute
1512 Gull Road
Kalamazoo, MI 49048
USA

Thierry Lefèvre MD
Interventional Cardiologist and
Head, Catheter Laboratory
Institut Hospitalier Jacques Cartier
Massy
FRANCE

Martin B Leon MD
President & CEO
Cardiovascular Research Foundation
New York, NY
USA

Jurgen M Ligthart BSc
Thoraxcenter, Erasmus Medical Center
Rotterdam
PO Box 2040
3000 CA Rotterdam
THE NETHERLANDS

Soo-Teik Lim
National Heart Centre of Singapore
Mistri Wing
17 Third Hospital Avenue
SINGAPORE 168752

Yean-Leng Lim
Director
Raffles Heart Centre
SINGAPORE

Joseph P Lindsay Jr MD
Chairman, Department of Cardiology
Washington Hospital Center
Washington, DC
USA

Talib K Majwal MD FRCPI FACC
Director, Interventional Cardiology
Department
Iraqi Center for Heart Disease
Baghdad
IRAQ

Carlo Di Mario
Catheterization Laboratory
Royal Brompton Hospital
Sydney Street
London SW3 6NP
UK

Winston Martin
Cardiology Department
University Hospital
Geneva
SWITZERLAND

Luiz Alberto Mattos MD PhD
Staff, Interventional Cardiology
Institute Dante Pazzanese of Cardiology
Sao Paulo
BRAZIL

Haresh Mehta
Consultant Cardiologist
PD Hinduja National Hospital and Medical
Research Center
Mumbai
INDIA

Bernhard Meier MD FACC FESC
Professor and Head of Cardiology and
Chairman, Swiss Cardiovascular Center
University Hospital
Bern
SWITZERLAND

Piero Montorsi MD
Interventional Cardiologist
Director, Clinical Cardiology
Institute of Cardiology
University of Milan
Centro Cardiologico Monzino IRCCS
Milan
ITALY

Marie-Claude Morice MD FESC FACC
Interventional Cardiologist
Head, Institut Cardiovasculaire Paris Sud
Paris
FRANCE

Jeffrey W Moses MD
Chief, Interventional Cardiology
Lenox Hill Heart and Vascular Insititute
New York, NY
USA

Christoph K Naber
Department of Cardiology
University of Essen
Essen
GERMANY

Eugenia Nikolsky
Division of Invasive Cardiology
Rambam Medical Center and
Technion – Israel Institute of Technology
Haifa
ISRAEL

Steven E Nissen MD FACC
Professor of Medicine and
Vice-Chairman, Department of Cardiovascular
Medicine
The Cleveland Clinic Foundation
Cleveland, OH
USA

Martin Oberhoff MD
Consultant Senior Lecturer in Cardiology
Bristol Heart Institute
University of Bristol
Bristol Royal Infirmary
Bristol
UK

xvi

Olaf Oldenburg MD
Fellow, Department of Cardiology
University Hospital of Essen
Essen
GERMANY

Michele Opizzi
Department of Anaesthesiology
San Rafaelle Hospital
Milan
ITALY

Serge Osula MRCPI
Consultant Cardiologist
North Cheshire Hospital Trusst
Warrington
UK

Jan Paul Ottervanger MD PhD
Consultant Cardiologist
ISALA Klinieken
Hospital De Weezenlanden
Zwolle
THE NETHERLANDS

Julio Palmaz MD
University of Texas HSC
at San Antonio
San Antonio, TX
USA

Seung-Jung Park MD PhD FACC
Professor of Medicine
Director, Interventional Cardiology
University of Ulsan College of Medicine
Cardiac Center
Asan Medical Center
Seoul
SOUTH KOREA

Chanderashekar V Patil MD
Division of Invasive Cardiology
Rambam Medical Center and Faculty of
Medicine
Technion – Israel Institute of Technology
Haifa
ISRAEL

Ian M Penn MBBS FRACP FRCP FESC
Director of Interventional Cardiology
Vancouver Hospital & Health Sciences Centre
865 West 10th Avenue
Vancouver BC V5Z 1L7
CANADA

Ibraim Pinto MD PhD
Director, Angiography Core Lab
Institute Dante Pazzanese of Cardiology
Sao Paulo
BRAZIL

David R Ramsdale FRCP MD
Consultant Cardiologist and
Director,
The Cardiothoracic Centre
Liverpool
UK

Evelyn Regar MD
Thoraxcenter
University Hospital Dijkzigt
Rotterdam
THE NETHERLANDS

Benno J Rensing MD
Department of Cardiology
St Antonius Hospital Nieuwegein
Koekoekslaan 1
3435 CM Nieuwegein
THE NETHERLANDS

Peter Ruygrok BSC MD FRACP FESC
Consultant Cardiologist
Green Lane Hospital
Auckland
NEW ZEALAND

Richard Schatz MD
Scripps Clinic and Research Foundation
La Jolla
California
USA

Pierre-Alain Schneider MD
Director, Invasive Radiology
Department of Cardiology
Hôpital de la Tour
Geneva
SWITZERLAND

Paul Schoenhagen MD FAHA
Fellow, Cardiovascular Tomography
Department of Cardiovascular Medicine and
Radiology
The Cleveland Clinic Foundation
Cleveland, OH
USA

Patrick Schopfer MD
Cardiologist
Department of Cardiology
Hôpital de la Tour
Geneva
SWITZERLAND

Patrick W Serruys
Thoraxcenter
University Hospital Dijkzigt
Rotterdam
THE NETHERLANDS

ACS Silva MD
Staff, Clinical Cardiology
Institute Dante Pazzanese of Cardiology
Sao Paulo
BRAZIL

Elliot Smith MBBS BSC MRCP
Specialist Registrar in Cardiology
Manchester Heart Centre
Manchester Royal Infirmary
Manchester
UK

J Eduardo Sousa MD PhD
Director, Institute "Dante Pazzanese" de
Cardiologia
São Paulo
BRAZIL

Amanda GMR Sousa MD PhD
Director, Invasive Cardiology
Institute Dante Pazzanese of Cardiology
Sao Paulo
BRAZIL

Vassilis Spanos
Department of Cardiology
San Rafaelle Hospital
Milan
ITALY

Kostantinos S Spargias
Department of Cardiology
Vancouver Hospital & Health Sciences Centre
865 West 10th Street
Vancouver BC
CANADA V5Z 1L7

Rodney H Stables
Consultant Cardiologist
The Cardiothoracic Centre
Liverpool
UK

R Staico MD
Staff, Clinical Cardiology
Institute Dante Pazzanese of Cardiology
Sao Paulo
BRAZIL

Goran Stankovic MD
Director, Cardiac Catheterization Laboratory
EMO Centro Cuore Columbus
Milan
ITALY

Harry Suryapranata MD PhD
Consultant Cardiologist and Director of
Clinical Research
ISALA Klinieken
Hospital De Weezenlanden
Zwolle
THE NETHERLANDS

Luiz Fernando Tanajura MD
Chief, Clinical Angioplasty
Institute Dante Pazzanese of Cardiology
Sao Paulo
BRAZIL

Daniela Trabattoni MD
Interventional Cardiologist
Institute of Cardiology
University of Milan
Centro Cardiologico Monzino IRCCS
Milan
ITALY

E Murat Tuzcu MD FACC
Professor of Medicine
IVUS Core Laboratory
Staff, Section of Interventional Cardiology
Department of Cardiovascular Medicine
The Cleveland Clinic Foundation
Cleveland, OH
USA

Philip Urban MD
Director, Interventional Cardiology
Department of Cardiology
Hôpital de la Tour
Geneva
SWITZERLAND

Stefan Verheye MD FESC
Interventional Cardiology
Cardiovascular Translational Research Institute
Department of Interventional Cardiology
Middelheim Hospital
Antwerp
BELGIUM

Renu Virmani MD
Chairman, Department of Cardiovascular
Pathology
Armed Forces Institute of Pathology
Washington, DC
USA

Alan Whelan MBChB FRACP
Interventional Fellow
Cardiology Department
Dunedin Hospital
Dunedin
NEW ZEALAND

Christopher J White MD
Chairman, Department of Cardiology
Ochsner Heart and Vascular Institute
Ochsner Clinic Foundation
New Orleans, LA
USA

Patrick L Whitlow MD FACC
Director, Interventional Cardiology
Department of Cardiovascular Medicine
The Cleveland Clinic Foundation
Cleveland, OH
USA

Gerard Wilkins MBChB FRACP
Cardiologist
Cardiology Department
Dunedin Hospital
Dunedin
NEW ZEALAND

Aaron Wong
National Heart Centre
SINGAPORE

Alan Yeung
Associate Professor of Medicine
Chief, Division of Cardiovascular Medicine
(Clinical)
Director, Cardiac Catheterization & Coronary
Intervention Laboratories
Stanford University Medical Center
Stanford, CA
USA

Felix Zijlstra
Cardiologist
Hospital De Weezenlanden
Zwolle
THE NETHERLANDS

PREFACE

Percutaneous coronary intervention is a continually evolving discipline. It is limited in its opportunity only by the technology and the experience of the operator. Case discussions and case review, from the beginning of intervention, have been the method of education, instruction and extension of an operator's experience. In every geographic location, case review meetings and live case demonstrations have become the medium of choice by which to evolve the specialty and an individual's understanding.

This book of selected cases has been compiled to facilitate education. Within these cases, we see examples of operators' innovating new solutions, extending the range of technology, often well outside the bounds of the 'indications for use' described by the manufacturer. However, as ever, the exceptional cases contributors describe today will become the norm of tomorrow. It is through case discussion that we see how to 'extend the envelope', and importantly, how not fall into the traps that others have experienced.

Through the medium of case discussion operators may develop new skills and avoid 'traps'. Tips and tricks are important for all of us to communicate to each other. The contributors to *Case Studies in Interventional Cardiology* are all highly experienced operators and communicators. The clarity of communication is obvious on every page and operators, experienced or 'novice', will benefit by the consideration of these case studies.

Martin T Rothman
London, 2003

GLOSSARY

ACEI	ACE (angiotensin-converting-enzyme) inhibitors
AF	atrial fibrillation
AMI	acute myocardial infarction
AP	angina pectoris
ASD	arterial septal defect
ASO	Amplatzer septal occluder (device)
BPG	base pressure gradient
CABG	coronary artery bypass graft
CASS	Coronary Artery Surgery Study
CBA	coronary balloon angioplasty
CK	creatine kinase
CPS	cardiopulmonary support
CFR	coronary flow reserve
CS	conventional stenting
CSA	cross-sectional area
CSS	Canadian Cardiovascular Society
CSSS	coronary–subclavian steal syndrome
CTO	chronic total occlusion
(L)Cx	(left) circumflex
D2	second diagonal branch
DCA	directional coronary atherectomy
DOE	dysnea on exertion
DS	direct stenting
ECG	electrocardiogram
EEM	external elastic membrane
EF	ejection fraction
ELCA	excimer laser coronary atherectomy
ELUTES	EvaLuation of Taxol-Eluting Stent
FDA	Food and Drug Administration
FFR	fractional flow reserve
Fr	French
H&E	h(a)ematoxylin eosin
HDL	high-density lipoprotein
HIT	heparin induced thrombocytopenia
HPG	hyper(a)emic pressure gradient
HSRA	high-speed rotational atherectomy
IABP	intraaortic balloon pump

ICA	internal carotid artery
ICRT	intracoronary radiation therapy
IRA	infarct-related artery
IVUS	intravascular ultrasound
LAD	left anterior descending
LAO	left anterior oblique
LIMA	left internal mammary artery
LMCA	left main coronary artery
LMS	left main stem
LV	left ventricular
LVEDP	left vestricular end-diastolic pressure
LVH	left ventricular hypertrophy
MACE	major adverse coronary event
MB	myocardial band
MLA	minimum lumen (cross-sectional) area
MLD	minimal lumen diameter
MLD	minimal luminal diameter
MVD	multivessel disease
OM	obtuse marginal
OM1	first obtuse marginal
OMB	obtuse marginal branch
PA	pulmonary artery
PCA	percutaneous cardiopulmonary supports
PCI	percutaneous coronary intervention
PCW	pulmonary capillary wedge
PND	paroxysmal nocturnal dysnea
POBA	plain old balloon angioplasty
PTCA	percutaneous transluminal coronary angioplasty
PTFE	polytetrafluoroethene
PVD	peripheral vascular disease
RAO	right anterior oblique
RBBB	right bundle branch block
RCA	right coronary artery
RI	ramus intermedius
RIMA	right internal mammary artery
RPD	right posterior descending
RSO	right superior oblique
RV	right ventricular
SVG	saphenous vein graft
TEE	trans(o)esophagal echocardiogram
TIA	transient isch(a)emic attack
TnT	troponin T
UFH	unfractionated heperinization
VD	vessel disease

Case 1

Elective Treatment Of Unprotected Left Main Coronary Artery (LMCA) Stenosis With Directional Coronary Atherectomy (DCA) Without Stenting

Antonio Colombo and Goran Stankovic

Background

A 44-year-old man with a history of hypercholesterolemia, hypertension and a positive family history for coronary artery disease presented with an anterior wall myocardial infarction in April 2000. Cardiac catheterization demonstrated a 90% stenosis in the distal segment of the left anterior descending (LAD) coronary artery and the patient underwent successful percutaneous transluminal coronary angioplasty (PTCA). Since August 2000, the patient has had repeated episodes of exertional chest discomfort, which were relieved by nitrates.

Repeat coronary angiography was performed in September 2000 and revealed a 70% distal LMCA stenosis, as well as a 90% restenosis of a lesion in the distal LAD (Fig. 1.1). The left circumflex (LCx) and the right coronary artery (RCA) exhibited only mild irregularities, and faint collaterals were present from the RCA to the distal segment of the LAD. A left ventriculogram demonstrated normal left ventricular (LV) systolic function. DCA of the distal left main stenosis was chosen due to the eccentric nature of the lesion, and the proximity of the LAD and the LCx ostia.[1–3]

At the beginning of the procedure, heparin was given at a dose of 70 IU/kg. The patient's blood pressure was 120 mmHg and the heart rate was 64 beats per minute (bpm). Intraaortic balloon counterpulsation was inserted through the left femoral artery with an 8 French (Fr) sheath. A 6 Fr sheath in the right femoral artery was replaced with an 8 Fr angioplasty sheath, and an 8 Fr guiding catheter XB 3.5 (Cordis; Johnson & Johnson Co, Miami, FL) was used to cannulate the left main ostium. A 300 cm long

1

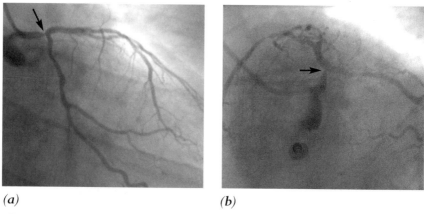

(a)   *(b)*

Figure 1.1 *Baseline coronary angiogram in the right anterior oblique (a) and the left anterior oblique – caudal projection (b) showing 70% stenosis of the distal left main coronary artery (arrows).*

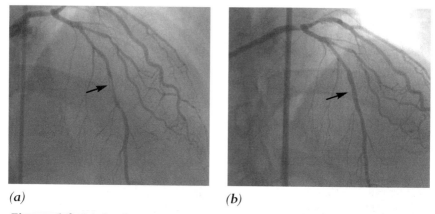

(a)   *(b)*

Figure 1.2 *(a) Baseline coronary angiogram in the right anterior oblique – cranial projection showing 90% stenosis of the distal left anterior descending coronary artery (arrow). (b) Final coronary angiogram in the same projection following direct coronary stenting, showing no residual stenosis (arrow).*

0.014 inch high-torque Iron Man wire (Guidant; Advanced Cardiovascular Systems, Inc, Temecula, CA) was advanced into the distal LAD. Direct stenting of the distal LAD restenotic lesion was performed using a Multi Link Tetra 3.0 × 18 mm stent (Guidant) (Fig. 1.2).

The next step was DCA of the LMCA stenosis. In this case, an 8 Fr compatible Flexi-cut 3.5–4 mm (Guidant) was selected. The lesion was treated by 10 passes of the cutter, while turning the device through 360° (Fig. 1.3). The post-procedure angiogram demonstrated a satisfactory result

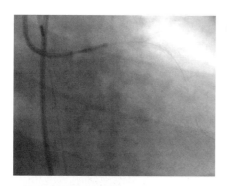

Figure 1.3. *Directional coronary atherectomy catheter (the Flexi-cut 3.5–4 mm, Guidant, Temecula, CA) positioned at the lesion site in the left main coronary artery.*

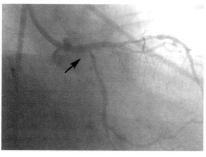

(a)

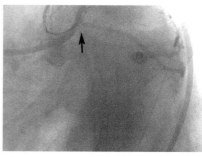

(b)

Figure 1.4 *Coronary angiogram in the right anterior oblique (**a**) and the left anterior oblique – caudal projection (**b**), following 10 passes of the atherectomy cutter, showing a satisfactory result without residual stenosis in the left main coronary artery but significant plaque shift into the ostial left circumflex coronary artery (arrows).*

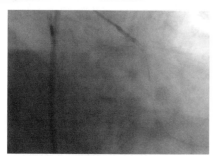

Figure 1.5 *Directional coronary atherectomy catheter (the Flexi-cut 3.5–4 mm, Guidant, Temecula, CA) positioned at the lesion site in the left circumflex coronary artery. Atherectomy was performed with six passes of the cutter.*

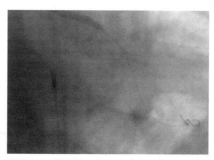

Figure 1.6 *Balloon angioplasty of the ostial left circumflex coronary artery performed following directional coronary atherectomy to optimize result.*

3

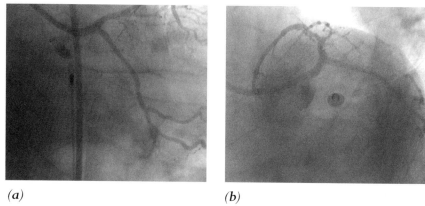

(a)   *(b)*

Figure 1.7 *Final coronary angiogram in the right anterior oblique (**a**) and the left anterior oblique − caudal projection (**b**), showing no significant residual stenosis in the distal left main coronary artery and ostium of the left circumflex coronary artery.*

without significant residual stenosis within the LMCA, but plaque shift into the ostial LCx was observed (Fig. 1.4). The guidewire was removed from the LAD and advanced into the LCx, and atherectomy of the ostial LCx was performed with six additional passes of the cutter (Fig. 1.5). Finally, the atherectomy device was exchanged for a balloon and angioplasty of the ostial LCx was performed to optimize results (Fig. 1.6). The final angiogram showed no significant residual stenosis (Fig. 1.7). The patient was free of angina, electrocardiographic change and/or hemodynamic instability.

The arterial sheath and the sheath of the balloon pump were removed immediately after the procedure, and a 6 Fr closure (Perclose, Inc, Redwood City, CA) device was used to achieve hemostasis. Further post-procedural outcomes were uneventful and the patient was discharged the following day, with the suggestion to continue ticlopidine and aspirin for 1 month, and then only aspirin.

Important considerations

Why DCA?

In bifurcational lesions, whenever possible, this group's preference is to do as much plaque debulking as possible. This proximal lesion was very suitable for this approach and follow-up results suggest that bifurcations effectively treated with debulking have good long-term outcomes.

Why stenting was not performed after DCA

Stenting was not performed after DCA because of the significant plaque shift, or new stenosis, in the LCx of the LMCA following this procedure – the LAD may predict a significant residual stenosis in the LCx following stenting of the LMCA toward the LAD. This assumption is made due to the fact that little material was retrieved when DCA was performed toward the LCx. This means that the narrowing of the LCx was most probably due to a change in the geometry of the angle of the LAD. Stenting of the LAD would have distorted this geometry, thus penalizing the LCx. The good final result obtained after DCA and balloon insertion gives a reasonable expectation for a low restenosis rate.

Why use a balloon pump?

Despite the fact this procedure was elective, this group favors temporary intraaortic balloon support while performing a debulking procedure on the LMCA. A balloon pump allows the operator to safely perform a more complete debulking procedure, minimizing patient discomfort. The possibility of using 8 Fr access in both groins and to immediately seal the entry sites with a 6 Fr suture-based closure device increases both the safety and tolerability of this procedure.

This patient, like everybody who undergoes a procedure on an unprotected LMCA, was scheduled for a routine angiographic follow-up 4–6 months following the procedure. The patient was also carefully instructed to report the occurrence not only of chest pain but also shortness of breath or fatigue, which may imply renarrowing of the LMCA.

References

1. Ellis SG, Tamai H, Nobuyoshi M et al. Contemporary percutaneous treatment of unprotected left main coronary stenoses: initial results from a multicenter registry analysis 1994–1996. *Circulation* 1997; **96**:3867–72.

2. Kosuga K, Tamai H, Ueda K et al. Initial and long-term results of angioplasty in unprotected left main coronary artery. *Am J Cardiol* 1999; **83**:32–7.

3. Silvestri M, Barragan P, Sainsous J et al. Unprotected left main coronary artery stenting: immediate and medium-term outcomes of 140 elective procedures. *J Am Coll Cardiol* 2000; **35**:1543–50.

Case 2

DIRECT LEFT MAIN TRUNK BIFURCATION STENTING IN ACUTE MYOCARDIAL INFARCTION (AMI)

David Antoniucci

Background

A 63-year-old man was admitted to our institution with anterior AMI and cardiogenic shock. Coronary angiography revealed a severe stenosis of the distal portion of the left main trunk with a TIMI grade 2 flow (Fig. 2.1). Direct stenting of the left main bifurcation using the 'V' technique was performed. Direct 'V' stenting was performed using two NIR stents (3.0/9 and 3.0/16 mm) which were delivered and expanded with a single simultaneous inflation at 16 atmospheres (Fig. 2.2). The post-procedure angiogram showed no residual stenosis and a TIMI grade 3 flow (Fig. 2.3). The 3- and 6-month follow-up angiography showed no restenosis of the treated lesion.

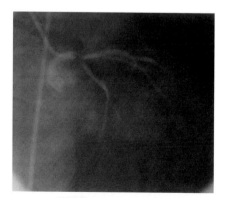

Figure 2.1. *Posteroanterior view showing left main bifurcation subocclusion.*

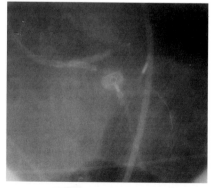

Figure 2.2. *Left caudal view showing kiss stenting ('V' stenting).*

7

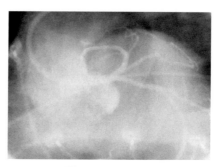

Figure 2.3. *Left caudal view showing final result.*

Commentary

Emergency left main trunk stenting

Stenting remains a challenging technique when the culprit lesion involves the origin of both branches of large bifurcations, such as the left main trunk bifurcation. In the setting of acute occlusion of the left main trunk complicated by AMI, the percutaneous technique approach requires a short procedural time, a maintained easy access to the left anterior descending (LAD) and circumflex (Cx) arteries, and a high probability of optimal acute angiographic result. The advent of low-profile, flexible last-generation stents has facilitated the access to side branches after stenting a main vessel. The coil stent bifurcation technique, as well as the 'T' stent technique, are relatively less demanding as compared to the 'Y' stent technique. However, crossing to the struts of an expanded stent with another stent remains a cumbersome procedure with the risk of an inappropriate position with regard to the ostium of the side branch ('T' stent technique), or insufficient scaffolding (coil stent technique). In patients with a left main bifurcation lesion, an emergency 'T' stenting technique could be considered when the Cx territory is not large and a possible failure of stenting of the ostium of the Cx artery would not be catastrophic. For these reasons, in the setting of left main bifurcation disease complicated by AMI, the 'V' stent technique may be considered the best stenting option, since this technique is technically less demanding, allows complete lesion coverage and the maintenance of access to both vessels.

Potential advantages of direct stenting (DS) in AMI

Primary infarct-related artery (IRA) stenting may be superior to conventional primary coronary angioplasty in patients with AMI.[1–5] Provisional IRA stent implantation improves the primary success rate, while elective stent implantation reduces the incidence of early and late IRA restenosis or reocclusion, and related cardiac events, mainly the need for repeat target vessel revascularization. However, completed randomized trials comparing primary IRA stenting and primary coronary angioplasty have shown no benefit of IRA stenting in terms of reduction of the incidence of angiographic no-reflow phenomenon, which is strongly related to mortality. In the Stent-PAMI trial, IRA stenting was associated with a trend toward a lower incidence of TIMI grade 3 flow at the end of the procedure and an increased mortality as compared to angioplasty alone.[5] On the other hand, an acute reduction of a normal angiographic flow after balloon angioplasty may be observed after stent deployment and expansion, suggesting that the negative effect on distal flow may be the consequence of increased atherosclerotic and thrombotic material embolization in the microvasculature. The rate of arterial embolization in the microvasculature after percutaneous coronary interventions (PCI) is unexpectedly high.[6] In patients with angina, the rate of arterial embolization complicated by myocardial infarction induced by stenting using a conventional technique appears to be greater than that occurring with balloon angioplasty.[7] It is likely that the pathological substrate of AMI, including an already disrupted atherosclerotic plaque with superimposed thrombosis, may potentiate the bulk atherosclerotic-platelet embolization promoted by catheter-based reperfusion therapy. DS could be expected to reduce embolization of plaque constituents and the incidence of the no-reflow phenomenon, thereby increasing perfusion and myocardial salvage in patients with AMI. It has been hypothesized that with the conventional stenting (CS) technique, the single or multiple high-pressure balloon inflations after stent deployment, associated with a bulky effect of the expanding stent, may promote the embolization of atherosclerotic debris and thrombotic material extruded through the struts during initial stent expansion.[5] Moreover, in animal models it has been shown that stent deployment and expansion with a single balloon inflation is associated with less vessel wall injury,[8] and, as a consequence, one may infer, less disruption to distal flow produced by embolic material. Finally, coronary angioscopy performed after direct stent implantation in patients with AMI, has shown that the stent exerts a 'jailing' effect on thrombotic material (Guagliumi G, personal communication Endovascular Therapies Course, Paris, May 2000). Potential disadvantages of the DS technique are embolization promoted during target lesion crossing attempt, stent loss, and incomplete balloon and stent expansion in a 'hard' calcified lesion. Enhanced designs of second-generation stents and delivery systems, as well as the enhanced crimping techniques, seem to overcome

9

these potential limitations, while the risk of an undilatable lesion in the setting of AMI may be considered remote.

DS was associated with a decreased incidence of no-reflow phenomenon as compared to CS in a series of 310 consecutive patients with AMI.[9]

References

1. Antoniucci D, Santoro GM, Bolognese L et al. A clinical trial comparing primary stenting of the infarct-related artery with optimal primary angioplasty for acute myocardial infarction. *J Am Coll Cardiol* 1998; **31**:1234–9.

2. Rodriguez A, Bernardi V, Fernandez M et al. In-hospital and late results of coronary stents versus conventional balloon angioplasty in acute myocardial infarction (GRAMI trial). *Am J Cardiol* 1998; **81**;1286–91.

3. Suryapranata H, van't Hof AWJ, Hoorntje JCA et al. Randomized comparison of coronary stenting with balloon angioplasty in selected patients with acute myocardial infarction. *Circulation* 1998; **97**:2502–5.

4. Saito S, Hosokawa G, Tanaka S, Nakamura S. Primary stent implantation is superior to balloon angioplasty in acute myocardial infarction: final results of the Primary Angioplasty versus Stent Implantation in Acute Myocardial Infarction (PASTA) trial. *Cathet Cardiovasc Intervent* 1999; **48**:262–8.

5. Grines CL, Cox DA, Stone GW et al. Coronary angioplasty with or without stent implantation for acute myocardial infarction. *N Engl J Med* 1999; **341**:1949–56.

6. Topol EJ, Yadav JS. Recognition of the importance of embolization in atherosclerotic vascular disease. *Circulation* 2000; **101**:570–80.

7. EPISTENT Investigators. Randomised controlled trial to assess safety of coronary stenting with use of abciximab. *Lancet* 1998; **352**:85–90.

8. Rogers C, Parikh S, Seifert P et al. Remnant endothelium after stenting enhances vascular repair. *Circulation* 1996; **94**:2909–14.

9. Moschi G, Migliorini A, Trapani M et al. Direct stenting without predilation in acute myocardial infarction. *Eur Heart J* 2000; **21**:525 (abstract).

Case 3

Left Main Stenosis Kept Simple

Stephen Ellis

Background

MR is a 90-year-old female transferred to our institution following presentation for the second time with congestive heart failure. Her cardiac history, other than mild hypertension, began only 3 weeks earlier when she presented to an outside hospital with dyspnea on exertion, noted over the previous 2 weeks. An electrocardiogram (ECG) and cardiac enzymes showed no evidence of myocardial infarction, and a chest X-ray showed severe pulmonary congestion. She was treated with diuretics and IV nitroglycerin. Following echocardiography, which revealed left ventricular hypertrophy (LVH) and normal systolic function, she underwent cardiac catheterization which revealed a 70% distal left main stenosis, diffuse 80–90% mid-left anterior descending coronary artery (LAD) stenosis and a subtotal occlusion of a heavily calcified mid-right coronary artery (RCA). The latter stenosis was successfully treated using a 3.0 × 50 mm S670 stent, leaving a 10% residual stenosis. The patient was discharged on aspirin, Tenormin 25 mg daily, Norvasc 5 mg daily, Plavix 75 mg daily and Dyazide.

One week following discharge, the patient had recurrent shortness of breath after a short walk and was readmitted to the outside community hospital. Cardiac enzymes were again negative. The ECG was unchanged, but the chest X-ray again showed pulmonary congestion. Following stabilization and initial treatment with diuretics and IV nitroglycerin, she was transferred to our institution for further care.

Upon arrival, further past medical history was obtained, which was notable for the fact that the patient was largely self-sufficient and lived alone, she did not have diabetes, pulmonary, renal or other major organ disease, and her father had passed away from a stroke. Cardiac enzymes remained negative. She was stabilized clinically and a referral for possible bypass surgery was obtained. Following discussion with the surgeons, the patient declined surgery due to concerns about the possibility of a cerebral vascular accident.

Repeat catheterization (Fig. 3.1a–c) revealed a good stent result in the RCA, albeit with diffuse disease, as well as the aforementioned distal left

11

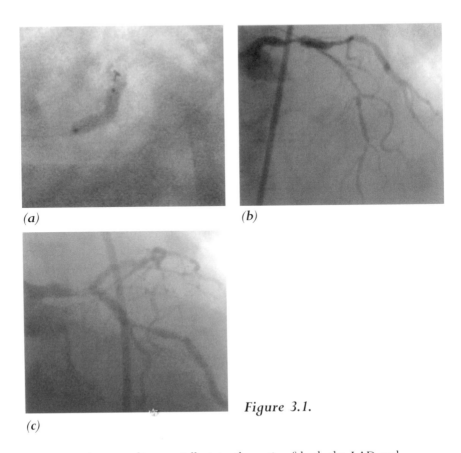

(a)

(b)

(c)

Figure 3.1.

main stenosis, extending partially into the ostia of both the LAD and circumflex (Cx) arteries, very severe and diffuse LAD disease, and a focal 70% narrowing in the obtuse marginal branch of the Cx.

Bearing in mind that there were several percutaneous options for treating the left main stenosis, but wishing to keep the procedure as simple and risk free as possible in this 90-year-old lady, we decided to place a single stent distally in the left main traversing into the LAD and to finish with kissing-balloon angioplasty in both the LAD and the Cx. We rejected the idea of debulking with rotational atherectomy, feeling that it was of unproven value and might increase the risk of non-Q-wave myocardial infarction. We also rejected the idea of 'T' or Coulette stenting because of the heightened risk of restenosis. Integrilin was used as the glycoprotein IIb/IIIa inhibitor complementary to aspirin and heparin. We did check the left ventricular end-diastolic pressure (LVEDP) prior to the procedure (20 mmHg) and afterwards (18 mmHg), but chose not to place a Swan–Ganz catheter or intraaortic balloon pump because of the heightened risk of complications in this frail lady. The procedure itself was performed with a 7 French (Fr)

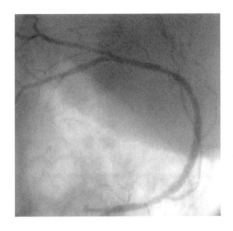

Figure 3.2.

(Judkins left 4) short-tipped Cordis guide, short Patriot guidewires down both the LAD and the Cx, predilatation using a 3.0 × 20 mm Adante balloon for both the LAD and the Cx, and stenting was accomplished using a 3.0 × 18 mm S670 stent (to provide reasonable side-branch access if needed). No attempt was made to treat the diffusely diseased LAD or Cx with the hope that a successful procedure would render this patient free of her recurrent pulmonary edema. The final technical result was acceptable (Fig. 3.2) and an 8 Fr Angio-Seal was deployed in the right femoral artery without complications. She was monitored in the intensive care unit overnight, the peak creatine kinase (CK) myocardial band (MB) was 6 and the patient was discharged 2 days later on aspirin, Plavix, Isordil, Norvasc, Lopressor, Hydralazine, Lasix and prn nitroglycerin.

The patient was seen in follow-up 2 months later, at which time cardiac catheterization had been recommended, but the patient declined due to her age. She had no subsequent cardiac symptoms with limited activity and she had remained independently active and able to care for herself.

Discussion

This case illustrates one approach to the technically challenging problem of percutaneous treatment of unprotected left main coronary disease. Increasing experience with this type of intervention has allowed us to understand better its current indications: (a) in the highly symptomatic but surgically inoperable patient; (b) in the patient presenting with acute myocardial infarction (AMI) and left main stenosis/occlusion;[1] (c) possibly in the low-risk patient (age

13

<65 years) left ventricular (LV) ejection fraction (EF) >40%, relatively focal left main stenosis who desires to avoid surgery. However, due to the risk of later sudden death (5–10% at 1 year), routine angiography is recommended at 2 and 6 months.[2,3]

References

1. Marso SP, Steg G, Plokker T et al. Catheter-based reperfusion of unprotected left main stenosis during an acute myocardial infarction (the ULTIMA experience). *Am J Cardiol* 1999; **83**:1513–17.

2. Ellis SG, Tamai H, Nobuyoshi M et al. Contemporary percutaneous treatment of unprotected left main coronary stenosis – initial results from a multicenter registry analysis 1994–96. *Circulation* 1997; **96**:3867–72.

3. Tan WA, Tamai H, Park S-J et al. for the ULTIMA Investigators. Long-term clinical outcomes after unprotected left main trunk percutaneous revascularization in 279 patients. *Circulation* 2001; **104**:1609–14.

Case 4

Unprotected Left Main Coronary Artery (LMCA) Stenting In A Young Female

Talib K Majwal

Background

The patient was a 26-year-old married female, mother of two children and a non-smoker. There was no history of hypertension or diabetes mellitus and her serum lipid profile was normal.

The patient was admitted to a general hospital with sudden onset of severe chest pain and electrocardiogram (ECG) changes of 2 mm ST-segment depression in the anterior leads, 2 weeks prior to her referral to our department.

Angiographic commentary

Emergency coronary angiography revealed severe distal LMCA stenosis prior to the bifurcation (Fig. 4.1), normal left anterior descending (LAD), left circumflex (LCx) and right coronary (RCA) arteries. Left ventricular (LV) ejection fraction (EF) was 62%. Intravascular ultrasound (IVUS) study showed soft atheroma in the distal LMCA not involving the ostia of the LAD or LCx (Fig. 4.2). The minimal luminal diameter (MLD) was 2.7 mm and the cross-sectional area (CSA) 6.7 mm^2.

An intraaortic balloon counter pulsation device was placed, but not used, prophylactically.

A 6 French (Fr) Judkins left 3.5 Vista bright-tip guiding catheter (Cordis Corp., Miami Lakes, FL) and a Wisdom 0.014 inch guidewire was advanced to the LAD. Since there was no extension of the atheroma to the LCx, no second wire for LCx protection was used. After predilation with a 3.0 mm balloon, immediate recoil occurred (Fig. 4.3). IVUS-guided stenting of the LMCA with a 4.0 × 8 mm Bx Velocity stent (Cordis) was undertaken and

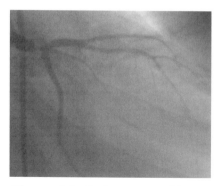

Figure 4.1. *Right anterior oblique (RAO) projection, showing severe distal left main stem coronary stenosis before the bifurcation.*

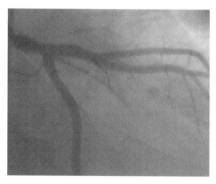

Figure 4.2. *IVUS, pre-intervention, soft atheroma, MLD = 2.7 mm and CSA = 6.7 mm².*

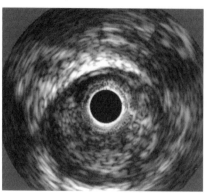

Figure 4.3. *Recoil after 3.0 mm balloon dilation.*

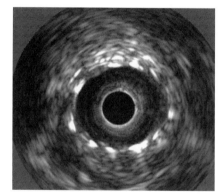

Figure 4.4. *RAO projection: good result after stenting with a 4.5 × 8 mm stent.*

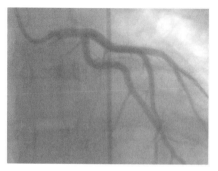

Figure 4.5. *Six months follow-up angiography showing patent stent, no evidence of restenosis.*

postdilated with a 4.5 mm balloon. A good result (Fig. 4.4) was achieved. Post-stenting IVUS (Fig. 4.5) shows a well-expanded stent, with an MLD of 4.6 mm and a CSA of 14.6 mm^2.

The patient was kept on ASA 325 mg and clopidogrel 75 mg daily, and discharged well the next morning.

At 6 months follow-up the patient was stable and asymptomatic, and angiography showed a patent stent with no evidence of restenosis.

This patient was number 57 to undergo stenting of an unprotected LMCA stenosis in our center over the last 2 years.

Case 5

The Unprotected Left Main Coronary Artery (LMCA) – A New Frontier For Angioplasty?

Marie-Claude Morice and Rajpal K Abhaichand

Background

Mr LJ, a 69-year-old male, a smoker and hypertensive, presented with unstable angina that was refractory to medical therapy. He had been operated on 6 months previously for invasive laryngeal carcinoma and had obstructive airway disease with a poor respiratory reserve. He continued to have rest pain on IV nitroglycerin, aspirin and heparin. During pain he had global ST-segment depression and, on one occasion, this was accompanied by pulmonary edema. He was referred to us for emergent coronary angiography and possible revascularization.

Angiographic commentary

Coronary angiography revealed a distal, eccentric, calcific 90% lesion of the LMCA that extended into and involved the proximal 10 mm of the left anterior descending (LAD) artery with a resultant 95% lesion (Fig. 5.1). The atheromatous plaque encompassed the left circumflex (LCx) ostium with a hemodynamically significant lesion. The large ramus intermedius (RI) was free of angiographic disease at its ostium, but had a tight lesion c. 2 cm after its origin. The right coronary artery (RCA) was dominant and free of disease. The clinical and angiographic findings were discussed with the cardiac surgery team and anesthesiologist, and it was felt that the patient was inoperable in view of his malignancy and poor respiratory reserve. After discussing the relevant issues with the patient, including the risk to life, it was decided to perform a high-risk percutaneous transluminal coronary angioplasty (PTCA) on this complex lesion.

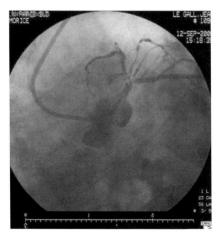 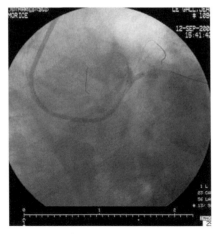

Figure 5.1. Diagnostic angiogram of the left coronary artery in the left anterior oblique view with a caudal projection, showing the complex lesion involving the distal left main, LAD and RI.

Figure 5.2. Angiogram showing that the trifurcation has been wired, and simultaneous deployment of stents in the ostial LAD and LCX.

The issues of concern were the unstable nature of the plaque and that it was a lesion involving the distal LMCA, with significant ostial LAD and LCx disease. The myocardium at risk was large and any further ischemia during the procedure would be poorly tolerated. Intraaortic balloon counterpulsation was electively instituted at the onset of the procedure, from the left groin. Once a Judkins left 4/8 French (Fr) guiding catheter was seated adequately in the ostium of the LMCA, the trifurcation was wired (Fig. 5.2) with three ACS Hi-torque balanced middleweight wires (Guidant; Europe SA). The proximal LAD and then the proximal RI were sequentially predilated with a 3 × 20 mm Viva balloon (Boston Scientific Corp.; Scimed). The proximal RI was then stented with a 3 × 13 mm Tetra stent (ACS; Guidant Corp.). Subsequently, two Bx Velocity stents (Cordis; Johnson and Johnson), 3 × 13 mm and 3 × 8 mm, were simultaneously deployed covering the ostia of the LAD and the LCx, respectively. As a result of plaque shift, the ostium of the RI was pinched and the segment immediately distal to the stented LAD was hazy. A short 3 × 8 mm stent was deployed adjacent to the first LAD stent. Subsequently, wires between the RI and the LAD were exchanged, i.e. the LAD wire was withdrawn into the LAD stent and passed into the RI through the strut of the LAD stent, and then the wire in the RI was used to wire the LAD. This was followed by a kissing inflation of three 3 × 20 mm Viva balloons at 10 atmospheres (Fig. 5.3). The wire in the RI was removed and then the LMCA

20

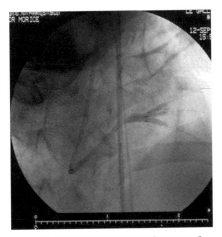

Figure 5.3. A kissing inflation of the trifurcation with three balloons.

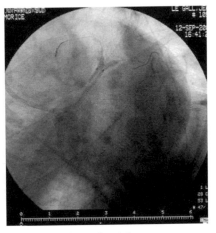

Figure 5.4. A final kissing inflation with balloons in the LAD and LCX arter stenting of the left main.

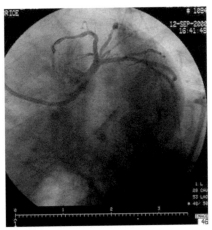

Figure 5.5. Final result after angioplasty of the left main and its trifurcation.

was stented with a 4.5 × 8 mm Tetra stent over the LAD wire. The wires in the LAD and the LCx were exchanged, and a final kissing dilatation was performed with two 3 mm Viva balloons at 10 atmospheres (Fig. 5.4). The results in the LMCA, the LAD and the LCx were excellent (Fig. 5.5), with minimal pinching of the RI, which was accepted.

Discussion

This case raises several issues of interest. Can we offer catheter-based therapy for unprotected left main lesions? Following the reduction in thrombotic complications after the introduction of ticlopidine therapy,[1-4] and the reduced rates of restenosis after stenting,[5,6] there is evidence to show that stent-supported angioplasty of the LMCA has a high rate of procedural success, with an acceptable morbidity and mortality.[7-9] Anatomically suitable lesions include those that clearly spare the distal LMCA at its bifurcation, up to moderately calcific lesions. Unsuitable lesions are those that involve the distal LMCA at the bifurcation and those which are densely calcific. We currently offer this therapy to all patients with anatomically suitable lesions and to those with distal bifurcation lesions who are at a high risk for coronary artery bypass surgery [i.e. left ventricular (LV) ejection fraction (EF) <35%, renal failure with serum creatinine kinase (CK) > 3 mg%, age > 75 years, poor distal vessels, inadequate respiratory reserve and other significant comorbid conditions that preclude surgery].

Is hemodynamic support mandatory? We now have restricted the use of intraaortic counterpulsation to patients presenting with cardiogenic shock, acute myocardial infarction (AMI) and those with complex distal lesions. Adequate operator experience, the use of a guiding catheter giving excellent support and rapid stent deployment are essential for procedural success. With both our experience with bifurcation disease[10] and that of others[9] we believe that distal left main bifurcation angioplasty is best completed with a kissing-balloon inflation as described above, to ensure a favorable immediate outcome and to reduce the incidence of restenosis.

What is the role of intravascular ultrasound (IVUS) in this setting? We performed IVUS after the LMCA stent was judged to be well deployed by angiography and in 72% of cases this led to the use of a bigger balloon dilatation, by c. 1 mm in diameter.[11] In this study, the target vessel revascularization at 15 months follow-up was 11%, with no cardiac death. We routinely perform IVUS in these patients, in order to optimize the minimal luminal diameter (MLD), usually to 0.5 mm more than the measured quantitative coronary angiographic or visually-assessed diameter.

Should the '6-month angiographic follow-up' dictum be followed? Since the incidence of restenosis of the LMCA is significant and can result in sudden cardiac death, we perform follow-up angiography at 2–4 months to detect restenosis, and either recommend surgery or perform a repeat angioplasty.

References

1. Barragan P, Sainsous J, Silvestri M et al. Ticlopidine and subcutaneous heparin as an alternative regimen following coronary stenting. *Cathet Cardiovasc Diagn* 1994; **32**:133–8.

2. Barragan P, Sainsous J, Silvestri M et al. Coronary artery stenting without anticoagulation, aspirin, ultrasound guidance, or high balloon pressure: prospective study of 1,051 consecutive patients. *Cathet Cardiovasc Diagn* 1997; **42**:367–73.

3. Karillon GJ, Morice MC, Benveniste E et al. Intracoronary stent implantation without ultrasound guidance and with replacement of conventional anticoagulation by antiplatelet therapy. Thirty-day clinical outcome of the French multicenter registry. *Circulation* 1996; **94**:1519–27.

4. Schoemig A, Neumann FJ, Kastrati A et al. A randomized comparison of anticoagulation and antiplatelet therapy after the placement of coronary stents. *N Engl J Med* 1996; **334**:1084–9.

5. Serruys PW, De Jaeger P, Kiemeneij F et al. A comparison of balloon expandable stent implantation with balloon angioplasty in the treatment of coronary artery disease. *N Engl J Med* 1994; **331**:489–95.

6. Fischman DL, Leon MB, Baim DS et al. A randomized comparison of coronary stent placement and balloon angioplasty in the treatment of coronary artery disease. *N Engl J Med* 1994; **331**:496–501.

7. Park SJ, Park SWS, Mong MK et al. Stenting of unprotected left main coronary artery stenosis. Immediate and late outcomes. *J Am Coll Cardiol* 1998; **31**:37–42.

8. Wong P, Wong V, Chan W et al. A prospective study of elective stenting in unprotected left main coronary disease. *Cathet Cardiovasc Intervent* 1999; **46**:153–9.

9. Silvestri M, Barragan P, Sainsous J et al. Unprotected left main coronary artery stenting: immediate and medium term-outcomes of 140 elective procedures. *J Am Coll Cardiol* 2000; **35**:1543–50.

10. Lefèvre T, Louvard Y, Morice MC et al. Stenting of bifurcation lesions: classification, treatments and results. *Cathet Cardiovasc Intervent* 2000; **49**:274–83.

11. Gobeil JF, Morice MC, Lefèvre T et al. Is intravascular ultrasound necessary for unprotected left main coronary angioplasty? *Eur Heart J* 2000; **21**:382(S).

Case 6

DEBULKING ATHERECTOMY IN BIFURCATION LEFT MAIN DISEASE

Seung-Jung Park

Background

A 50-year-old man was referred for recent-onset minimal effort angina. The risk factors for coronary artery disease were recently detected diabetes mellitus and the history of 30 pack-years smoking. The electrocardiogram showed T-wave inversion at lateral leads. The echocardiography revealed a normal left ventricular (LV) contractility without regional wall motion abnormalities.

Angiographic commentary

The left coronary angiogram showed tight stenoses along the entire length of the left main stem, and the ostium of the left anterior descending (LAD), the left circumflex (LCx) and intermediate arteries (Fig. 6.1.) Directional coronary atherectomy (DCA) [7 French (Fr)] was performed prior to stenting in the left main and into the LAD (Fig. 6.2a) and LCx (Fig. 6.2b) arteries, respectively.

After DCA, the coronary angiogram showed improved perfusion at the lesion sites (Fig. 6.3).

Left main stenting was performed with a 4.0 × 9 mm NIR stent (Fig. 6.4).

After main stenting, kissing stenting was performed at the ostium of the LAD and the ostium of the LCx with two 4.0 × 9 mm premounted NIR stents (Fig. 6.5). After stenting at the left main, the LAD and the LCx arteries, the coronary angiogram showed near normal coronary perfusion at the lesion sites (Fig. 6.6).

A 6-month angiogram showed widely patent NIR stents at the left main bifurcation site with minimal narrowing at the ostium of the left LCx and obtuse marginal artery (Fig. 6.7).

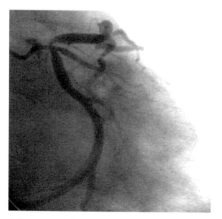

Figure 6.1.

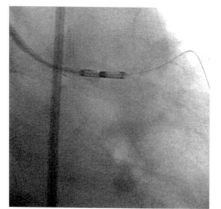

Figure 6.2a.

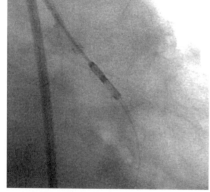

Figure 6.2b.

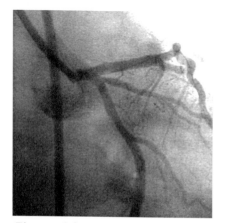

Figure 6.3.

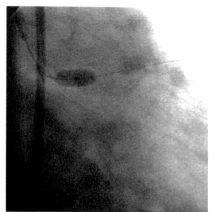

Figure 6.4.

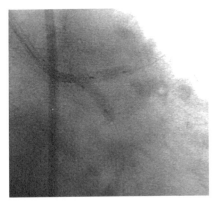

Figure 6.5.

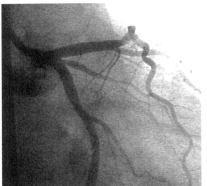

Figure 6.6.

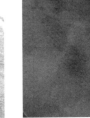

Figure 6.7.

Discussion

The bulk of the atheromatous plaque is displaced, but not removed, by balloon angioplasty, limiting complete stent expansion. By removing the plaque, DCA may facilitate successful stent placement. A recent study showed that, like non-stented lesions, residual plaque burden was also an important predictor of intimal hyperplasia in stented lesions.[1] The authors suggested that aggressive debulking with DCA before stenting might reduce the residual plaque burdens and, subsequently, the restenosis.[2] This approach may be especially useful for treatment of distal left main coronary artery (LMCA) stenosis because debulking atherectomy can improve the initial results of stenting.

From November 1995 to April 2000, 127 consecutive patients with unprotected LMCA stenosis and normal LV function were treated with elective stenting at Asan Medical Center. Debulking procedures with DCA before stenting were performed in 40 lesions during the later study period. Optimal atherectomy and adjunct balloon angioplasty was performed in all 40 cases until the residual diameter was <10% by visual estimate. Compared with stenting alone, the debulking plus stenting approach had a significantly lower rate of angiographic restenosis (8.3 versus 25.0%, $P = 0.034$). Serial IVUS comparison of pre-intervention and post-DCA at the same pre-intervention lesion site was performed in 24 of 30 lesions with DCA plus stenting. The plaque burden decreased from 86 to 55% and luminal diameter increased from 2.6 $\pm$ 0.9 to 8.9 $\pm$ 2.0 mm^2 after DCA. The reduction of plaque was 30%; the plaque plus media cross-sectional area (CSA) decreased from 19.9 $\pm$ 6.5 to 12.1 $\pm$ 5.6 mm^2.

References

1. Prati F, Di Mario C, Moussa I et al. In-stent neointimal proliferation correlates with the amount of residual plaque burden outside the stent: an intravascular ultrasound study. *Circulation* 1999; **99**:1011–14.

2. Moussa I, Moses J, Mario CD et al. Stenting after optimal lesion debulking (SOLD) registry. Angiographic and clinical outcome. *Circulation* 1998; **98**:1604–9.

Case 7

LEFT MAIN DISSECTION DURING PRIMARY ANGIOPLASTY FOR ACUTE MYOCARDIAL INFARCTION (AMI)

Jan Paul Ottervanger and Harry Suryapranata

Case presentation

A 52-year-old patient was included in our Pre-Hospital Infarct Angioplasty Triage protocol, using computer-assisted myocardial infarct diagnosis by 12-lead electrocardiogram (ECG) made in the ambulance.[1] He was admitted to the hospital complaining of substernal pain accompanied by nausea and vomiting, starting 1 hour before admission. His medical history revealed diabetes mellitus, which was treated with oral antidiabetics, and he also had a family history of coronary heart disease.

Upon admission, the patient was normotensive (systolic blood pressure 120 mmHg), had normal peripheral pulses and had no signs of congestive heart failure. The ECG showed a regular sinus rhythm of 76 beats/min with a normal PQ interval. However, in leads V1–V4, elevation of the ST segment was seen, accompanied by inverted T-waves in leads V4, V6, I and AVL.

The patient was transported immediately to the catheterization laboratory. Angiography, performed via the right femoral artery, showed a significant stenosis in the posterolateral branch of the right coronary artery (RCA). In the left coronary artery (LCA), there was a non-significant lesion in the left anterior descending (LAD) artery, while a significant stenosis in the obtuse marginal branch (OMB) and a subtotally occluded posterolateral branch were observed (Fig. 7.1). Subsequently, primary angioplasty of the posterolateral branch was performed. However, after the first balloon inflation, a major dissection of the left main was observed, with occlusion of both the ramus circumflexus and the LAD (Fig. 7.2). The patient experienced severe chest pain and became hypotensive. As the guidewire was still in place, immediate stenting of the posterolateral branch of the circumflexus (target lesion) was performed. The guidewire was then removed from the circumflexus and reinserted into the LAD, followed by immediate stenting of the left main

29

(Fig. 7.3). This resulted in restoration of the blood flow in both LCA, with relief of chest pain and normalization of blood pressure. However, there was a suboptimal result of angioplasty (Fig. 7.4). An intraaortic balloon pump was then inserted and the patient was referred for urgent coronary bypass

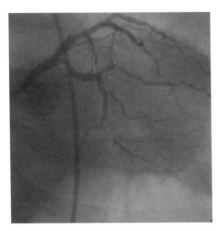

Figure 7.1. *Immediate angiogram showing a subtotally occluded postero-lateral branch while no significant stenosis is observed in the LAD.*

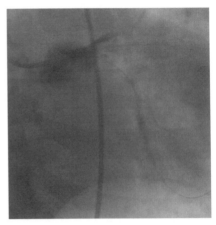

Figure 7.2. *Major dissection with occlusion of the left main after the first balloon inflation of the postero-lateral branch (target lesion of the infarct-related artery).*

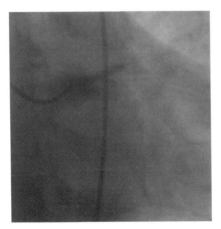

Figure 7.3. *Immediate stenting of the left main.*

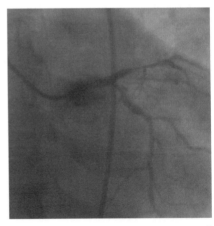

Figure 7.4. *Resulting restoration of antegrade flow, with relief of chest pain and normalization of blood pressure.*

surgery. Within 2 hours after the dissection, the left internal mammary artery (LIMA) was connected to the LAD and a vein jump graft on the obtuse marginal (OM), the left posterolateral and the right posterolateral branches. This resulted in only minimal creatine kinase (CK) myocardial bond (MB) release. The patient recovered uneventfully over the following days.

Discussion

Over the past few decades, the indications for angioplasty have increased and now include treatment of AMI. Although the beneficial results of primary angioplasty and stenting in patients with AMI have been demonstrated in randomized trials, this method of early reperfusion cannot be implemented in all settings. Over the past decade, primary angioplasty has been performed at our institution in a routine manner as the only reperfusion strategy for AMI.[2] The results have been reported in several journals and the long-term benefits of this strategy have recently been published.[3] In the 194 patients randomized to primary angioplasty in our study, urgent coronary artery bypass grafts (CABG) were necessary in seven patients (3.6%); the outcome of these patients was excellent. Other studies have shown that CABG may be necessary in up to 1.5% of patients with coronary angioplasty.[4] These results, together with the case described herein, imply that there remains a need for surgical standby, even in this era of stenting, and that the treatment of patients with AMI is not an 'all-or-nothing' scenario.

One of the potential complications of primary angioplasty is shown in this case. Although the need for urgent revascularization in our patient could be argued due to a small and patent infarct-related vessel, angioplasty was performed with, as a complication, dissection of the left main. However, as our patient had hardly any delay of reperfusion after the dissection of the left main, the occurrence of a large myocardial infarction was avoided. It has been said that cardiac surgery today is like the teddy bear of interventional cardiology; it is nice to have it around but, in fact, you don't really need it to sleep. However, it should not be forgotten that over the past decades, the continuing support of our 'big brothers' in cardiac surgery has led to rapid developments in interventional cardiology. Also, even more importantly, despite the fact that it has been demonstrated that the need for urgent surgery has been significantly reduced in the stenting era,[5,6] losing one patient due to the lack of surgical standby is one casualty too many.

The case reported here emphasizes the need for on-site cardiothoracic surgery. This is particularly necessary in primary angioplasty for AMI since the coronary anatomy is not known in these patients before angiography. In this situation, angioplasty is frequently performed in patients with multivessel disease (MVD) and who are haemodynamically unstable, and it therefore concerns a high-risk group. However, since it is difficult to predict accurately complications of angioplasty in an individual patient, in our opinion, on-site surgical backup is essential in every hospital in which coronary angioplasty is performed.

References

1.   Zijlstra F. Long-term benefit of primary angioplasty compared to thrombolytic therapy for acute myocardial infarction. *Eur Heart J* 2000; **21**:1487–9.

2.   De Boer MJ, Suryapranata H, Hoorntje JCA et al. Limitation of infarct size and preservation of left ventricular function after primary coronary angioplasty compared with intravenous streptokinase in acute myocardial infarction. *Circulation* 1994; **90**:753–61.

3.   Zijlstra F, Hoorntje JCA, de Boer MJ et al. Long-term benefit of primary angioplasty as compared with thrombolytic therapy for acute myocardial infarction. *N Engl J Med* 1999; **341**:1413–19.

4.   Andreasen JJ, Mortensen PE, Andersen LI et al. Emergency coronary artery bypass surgery after failed percutaneous transluminal coronary angioplasty. *Scand Cardiovasc J* 2000; **34**:242–6.

5.   Richie JL, Maynard C, Every NR et al. Coronary artery stent outcomes in a Medicare population: less emergency bypass surgery and lower mortality rates in patients with stents. *Am Heart J* 1999; **138**:437–40.

6.   Hannan EL, Racz MJ, Arani DT et al. A comparison of short- and long-term outcomes for balloon angioplasty and coronary artery stent placement. *J Am Coll Cardiol* 2000; **36**:395–403.

Case 8

CORONARY ARTERY PERFORATION AND HEMODYNAMIC COLLAPSE COMPLICATING STENT DEPLOYMENT: SUCCESSFUL MANAGEMENT WITH PERCUTANEOUS CARDIOPULMONARY SUPPORT (CPS) AND STENT GRAFT IMPLANTATION

Antonio L Bartorelli, Daniela Trabattoni and Piero Montorsi

Background

A 69-year-old man presented with exercise-induced anterolateral reversible perfusion defect 8 months after successful stenting of the left anterior descending (LAD) coronary artery.

Figure 8.1. *Left coronary artery (LCA) angiography in right anterior oblique (RAO) projection with cranial angulation. (**a**) Eccentric stenosis of the mid-LAD (arrow). Note the moderate restenosis of the previously implanted stent (arrowheads). (**b**) Moderate residual stenosis is seen after ACS Multi-Link RX Tristar stent deployment. (**c**) Short (12 mm) 3.5 mm diameter balloon inflated at high pressure (16 atmospheres) to fully expand the stent. (**d**) After balloon deflation, angiography demonstrates brisk dye extravasation due to free coronary perforation. Arrowheads denote the stent's ends. (**e**) After hemodynamic stabilization with CPS and prolonged balloon inflation, pulsatile dye extravasation is still evident. (**f**) Final angiography, demonstrating complete sealing of the LAD perforation with no evident contrast extravasation after JoMed graft stent implantation. Compared with the previous angiograms, occlusion of small septal and diagonal branches arising from the stent graft implantation site is evident.*

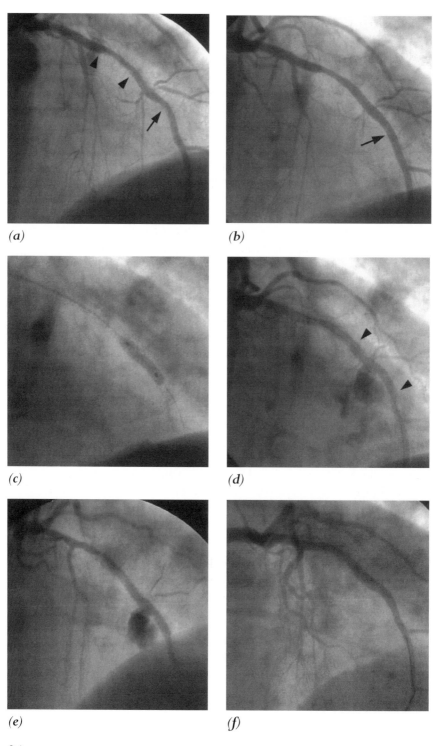

(a)

(b)

(c)

(d)

(e)

(f)

Angiographic commentary

Coronary angiography revealed patency with mild hyperplastic response of the previously implanted LAD stent and *de novo* eccentric stenosis of the mid-LAD (Fig. 8.1a). Direct stenting of the mid-LAD lesion was performed with an 18 mm long, 3.0 mm diameter Multi-Link RX Tristar stent (Guidant Advanced Cardiovascular Systems, Santa Clara, USA) deployed at 14 atmospheres. Angiography revealed incomplete stent expansion (Fig. 8.1b). Stent postdilation at 16 atmospheres was performed with a 12 mm long, 3.5 mm diameter Seajet non-compliant balloon (Nycomed Amersham Medical Systems, Paris Cedex, France) (Fig. 8.1c). Control angiography showed large coronary artery perforation at the stent implantation site with pulsatile contrast extravasation into the pericardium (Fig. 8.1d). Despite reinflation of the angioplasty balloon quickly performed at the site of contrast extravasation, the patient developed cardiac tamponade (Fig. 8.2a) and hemodynamic collapse. External cardiac massage was immediately started and pericardiocentesis was performed with a multiple-side-hole catheter, reinfusing the aspired blood in the patient. However, resuscitation maneuvers failed. Therefore, percutaneous cardiopulmonary support (CPS) was initiated through the right femoral vessels (Fig. 8.3), obtaining hemodynamic stabilization. At repeat angiography, performed after prolonged balloon inflation at the stent site, there was still evidence of free contrast extravasation into the pericardium through the LAD coronary artery perforation (Fig. 8.1e). Thus, the use of a JoStent coronary stent graft (JoMed International AB, Helsingborg, Sweden) was considered. This stent consists of two coaxially-aligned tubular stainless steel stents encompassing a microporous polytetrafluoroethylene (PTFE) membrane (75 µm) in a sandwich-like configuration (Fig. 8.4). The stent is available in lengths of 9, 12, 19 and 26 mm, and its potential diameter is 2.5–5.0 mm. A 12 mm long JoStent coronary stent graft was hand crimped on a 20 mm long, 3.5 mm diameter Worldpass balloon catheter (Cordis Medical Systems, Waterloo, Belgium), passed inside the previously placed Multi-Link stent, deployed at 14 atmospheres at the perforation site and postdilated at 18 atmospheres with a 12 mm long, 3.5 mm diameter Seajet balloon catheter (Nycomed Amersham Medical Systems, Paris, Cedex, France). Final angiography showed successful sealing of the coronary artery perforation (Fig. 8.1f). Pericardial effusion was no longer visible under 2D-echocardiographic control (Fig. 8.2b).

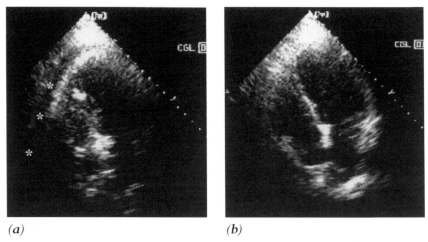

(a)   (b)

Figure 8.2. *Apical four-chamber 2D echocardiogram. (a) Large pericardial effusion with cardiac tamponade (*). (b) After pericardiocentesis, pericardial effusion is no longer present.*

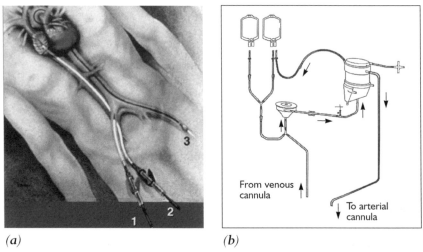

(a)   (b)

Figure 8.3. *(a) Percutaneous insertion of the arterial and venous CPS cannulae. The arterial cannula (1) was advanced to the proximal common iliac artery, while the venous cannula (2) was placed above the junction between the right atrium and the inferior vena cava. A left percutaneous approach (3) was used for graft stent implantation after hemodynamic stabilization of the patient. (b) Diagram of the CPS components and circuit. The venous blood is aspirated by a centrifugal pump, propelled through the heat exchanger and the membrane oxygenator and returned to the patients. Volume, crystalloid or blood products can be introduced through the priming line.*

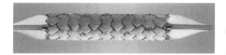

Figure 8.4. *The JoStent coronary stent graft. Sandwich technology integrates an ultrathin layer of expandable PTFE placed between two coaxially-aligned stainless steel tubular slotted stents.*

Discussion

The incidence of coronary artery perforation and/or rupture with percutaneous transluminal coronary angioplasty (PTCA) is as low as 0.14%,[1] but has shown a significant increase (0.25–3.0%) with the introduction of newer interventional devices such as stents, excimer laser angioplasty, directional atherectomy and rotablation.[2,3] The technique of high-pressure balloon dilation of the stented segment after stent deployment is commonly used to fully expand the stent, but it may cause vessel wall perforation by different mechanisms: (a) overdistension of the most compliant coronary artery segment; (b) high-pressure jet due to balloon rupture; (c) outward pushing of a stent strut through the vessel wall. In any of these cases, vessel calcification or intense fibrosis may increase the risk of perforation. Moreover, the stent's scaffolding effect and the heparin anticoagulation, with or without the use of glycoprotein IIb/IIIa inhibitors or platelet inhibitors, may keep the hole open and impede thrombus formation, causing unrelenting hemorrhage. Initial management of this serious complication includes prolonged balloon inflation at the site of contrast extravasation, eventually with the use of a perfusion balloon,[1–3] stent placement[4] and reversal of heparin anticoagulation with protamine administration.[5] However, in one-third of patients these simple measures fail and may even enlarge the arterial tear, causing further intrapericardial bleeding, rapid cardiac tamponade and cardiac arrest. When hemodynamic deterioration occurs, the management is focused on patient stabilization, pericardiocentesis and emergent surgery with the repair of the culprit vessel. In the present case, we used CPS to obtain hemodynamic stabilization after failure of conventional resuscitation maneuvers[6] and we managed the coronary artery perforation with an endovascular approach. PTFE-covered stent graft implantation is an easy and rapid alternative to surgery, which is more practical and may decrease the risk of death, especially in emergency situations. Case reports and small clinical series have shown promising results of the JoMed covered stent graft in the treatment of coronary artery perforation.[7–9] The main limitations of

37

this device are late thrombosis,[10] which could be prevented by high-pressure balloon inflation and intravascular ultrasound (IVUS) evaluation of proper implantation, limited trackability in tortuous and diffusely diseased vessels, and occlusion of side branches.

References

1. Alunji SC, Glazier S, Blakenship L et al. Perforations after percutaneous coronary interventions. Clinical, angiographic and therapeutic observations. *Cathet Cardiovasc Diagn* 1994; **32**:206–12.

2. Ellius SG, Ajluni S, Arnold AZ et al. Increased coronary perforation in the new device era: incidence, classification, management, and outcome. *Circulation* 1994; **90**:2725–30.

3. Holmes DR, Reeder GS, Ghazzal ZM et al. Coronary perforation after excimer laser coronary angioplasty: the excimer laser coronary angioplasty registry experience. *J Am Coll Cardiol* 1994; **23**:330–5.

4. Thomas MR, Wainwright RJ. Use of an intracoronary stent to control intrapericardial bleeding during coronary artery rupture complicating coronary angioplasty. *Cathet Cardiovasc Diagn* 1993; **30**:169–72.

5. Briguori C, Di Mario C, De Gregorio J et al. Administration of protamine after coronary stent deployment. *Am Heart J* 1999; **138**:64–8.

6. Shawl AF. Emergency percutaneous cardiopulmonary bypass support in patients with cardiac arrest. In: (Shawl FA, ed). *Supported Complex and High-risk Coronary Angioplasty.* (Kluwer Academic Publishers: Dordrecht, 1991) 145–65.

7. Ramsdale DR, Mushawar SS, Morris JL. Repair of coronary artery perforation after rotastenting by implantation of the JoStent covered stent. *Cathet Cardiovasc Diagn* 1998; **45**:310–13.

8. Casella G, Wemer F, Klauss V et al. Successful treatment of coronary artery perforation during angioplasty using a new membrane-coated stent. *J Invasive Cardiol* 1999; **11**:622–6.

9. Briguori C, Nishida T, Anzuini A et al. Emergency polytetrafluoroethylene-covered stent implantation to treat coronary ruptures. *Circulation* 2000; **102**:3028–31.

10. Elsner M, Auch-Schwelk W, Britten M et al. Coronary stent grafts covered by polytetrafluoroethylene membrane. *Am J Cardiol* 1999; **84**:335–8.

Case 9

TOTAL CORONARY OCCLUSION AND HYDROPHILIC GUIDEWIRES

Bruce R Brodie

Background

A 47-year-old man admitted with a non-Q-wave myocardial infarction underwent catheterization 1 day later and was found to have total occlusion of the circumflex (Cx) intermediate artery with minimal distal collaterals. He also had 90% stenosis in a small obtuse marginal branch (OMB), 50% stenosis in the proximal left anterior descending (LAD) artery and total occlusion of a small right coronary artery (RCA). The left ventriculogram showed inferior wall hypokinesis with an ejection fraction (EF) of 48%. Intervention was planned on the Cx intermediate artery.

Angiographic commentary

The procedure was performed with a 7 French (Fr) 3.5 Voda guiding catheter using weight-adjusted heparin to prolong the ACT to >200 seconds, and abciximab bolus and infusion. The lesion was crossed with some difficulty using a Cordis Shinobi hydrophilic wire, predilated and then stented with a 3.5 × 25 mm NIR stent, and postdilated with a 3.5 × 22 mm Ranger balloon as shown in the figures.

Two hours post-procedure, the patient developed hypotension and bradycardia not responsive to IV fluids, atropine and dopamine. Echocardiography demonstrated a pericardial effusion with tamponade. Abciximab was discontinued, platelets were ordered and the patient was taken urgently back to the catheterization laboratory for pericardiocentesis. Following pericardiocentesis and platelet transfusion his condition stabilized. The Cx intermediate artery was occluded and no attempt was made to reopen the artery. He was discharged home 2 days later in stable condition.

39

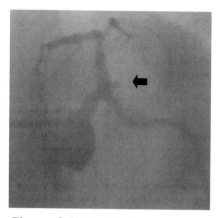

Figure 9.1. *The baseline image in the left anterior oblique (LAO); caudal projection shows total occlusion of the Cx intermediate artery (arrow).*

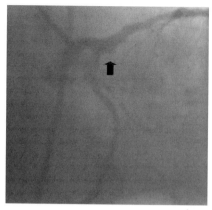

Figure 9.2. *The occlusion is shown in the right anterior oblique (RAO); caudal projection (arrow).*

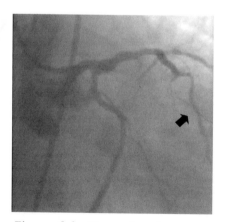

Figure 9.3. *The total occlusion could not be crossed with a soft floppy wire or an intermediate wire. A Cordis Shinobi hydrophilic wire was advanced distally but did not move freely, did not re-establish flow and a 2.0 × 20 mm Ranger balloon would not follow the wire. The wire was re-routed as shown and the distal tip then appeared to move freely.*

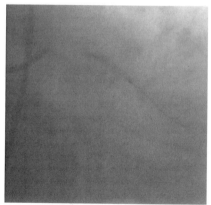

Figure 9.4. *A 2.0 × 20 mm Ranger balloon was inflated to 8 atmospheres.*

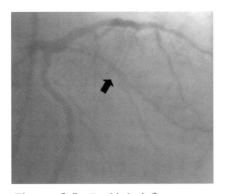

Figure 9.5. Established flow into the distal vessel.

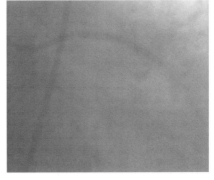

Figure 9.6. A 3.5 × 25 mm NIR stent was deployed at 15 atmospheres.

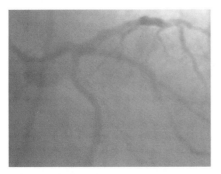

Figure 9.7. The post-stenting image showed a widely patent lumen.

Figure 9.8. The stent was further expanded with a 3.5 × 22 mm non-compliant Ranger balloon inflated to 18 atmospheres.

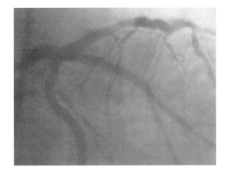

Figure 9.9. The final angiographic result showed a widely patent lumen at the stent site with moderate distal disease.

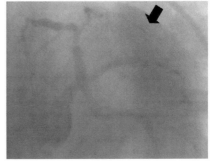

Figure 9.10. The final angiographic image in the LAO; caudal projection also shows a widely patent lumen. There was an unexplained density indicated by the arrow.

Figure 9.11.
The Cx intermediate artery has re-occluded at the stent site.

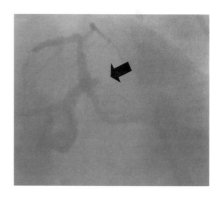

Discussion

This represents a case of unrecognized wire perforation resulting in pericardial tamponade 2 hours post-procedure. Hydrophilic wires, such as the Shinobi wire, are helpful in crossing total occlusions but are also associated with an increased risk of perforation. These wires should be used with caution and with diligent control of the distal tip. Usually, wire perforations do not cause serious sequelae; however, in the presence of glycoprotein IIb/IIIa platelet inhibition, wire perforations are less likely to seal and pericardial tamponade can occur. Except in the setting of acute coronary occlusion [acute myocardial infarction (AMI)] the use of glycoprotein IIb/IIIa platelet inhibitors as adjunctive therapy for intervention on a totally occluded coronary artery probably should be deferred until the lesion is crossed with the wire and it is certain that the distal tip of the wire is free in the true lumen.

Case 10

CORONARY ARTERY GUIDEWIRE PERFORATION DURING CORONARY INTERVENTION TREATED WITH LOCAL DELIVERY OF INTRACORONARY THROMBIN

Tim A Fischell, Michael Lauer and Malcolm T Foster

Background

The patient is an 86-year-old male who presented with clinical symptoms suggestive of unstable angina. He was admitted to the telemetry unit and ruled out for myocardial infarction by standard creatine kinase (CK) myocardial band (MB) criteria. The resting electrocardiogram (ECG) demonstrated minor T-wave flattening in the lateral leads, without other specific abnormalities. Physical examination was unremarkable, with the exception of scattered rales at the right lung base and a soft S4 apical gallop rhythm. He was referred for coronary angiography and possible coronary revascularization.

Angiographic commentary

The patient had selective coronary angiography which demonstrated: (a) a small non-dominant right coronary artery (RCA); (b) mild disease in the left anterior descending (LAD) coronary artery and (c) severe multifocal coronary disease involving the mid- and distal portion of the dominant left circumflex (LCx), and the proximal/ostial portion of a large first obtuse marginal (OM1) branch. The initial angiographic images of the LCx, prior to intervention, are shown in the right anterior oblique (RAO) and left anterior oblique (LAO) views (Figs 10.1 and 10.2, respectively). After reviewing the patient's anatomy, it was felt that the LCx and OM1 disease was the cause of the patient's clinical syndrome, and intervention was performed. Systemic heparin (8000 IU) and IV ReoPro (usual weight-adjusted bolus and drip) were administered. The left coronary was engaged using an 8 French (Fr) Judkins left 4 guiding catheter (Cordis Corp., Miami Lakes, FL). A two-wire technique was used and percutaneous transluminal coronary angioplasty (PTCA) followed by stenting was performed in the true LCx. After predilatation, a 3.0 × 16 mm length NIR stent was implanted distally and a 3.5 × 15 mm length Crown stent was placed more proximally in the true LCx. A Scimed, Graphix PT wire was used to cross the lesion in the OM1. After predilatation, a 2.75 × 15 mm Minicrown stent was placed at the ostial portion of the OM1. This caused some plaque shift into the main LCx. This was then treated with kissing-balloon angioplasty in the OM1 and the LCx, simultaneously, which achieved a good result (see Fig. 10.3). During this kissing-balloon manipulation it was appreciated that the distal tip of the Choice PT Graphix wire had broken off and embolized into the terminal portion of the OM1 branch (Fig. 10.3).

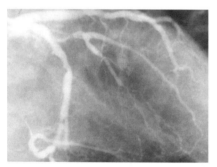

Figure 10.1. Angiogram in right anterior oblique (RAO) view, showing lesions in the true LCx and proximal obtuse marginal branch.

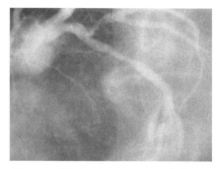

Figure 10.2. Angiogram in left anterior oblique (LAO) view, showing lesions in the true LCx and proximal obtuse marginal branch.

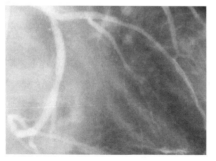

Figure 10.3. Angiogram in RAO view, showing result after stenting and angioplasty of true LCx and proximal obtuse marginal branch.

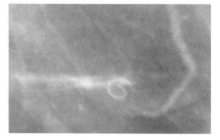

Figure 10.4. Magnified angiographic view showing contrast extravasation from distal guidewire perforation in obtuse marginal branch. Fractured fragment of guidewire tip is seen.

44

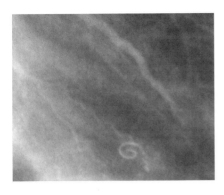

Figure 10.5. Magnified angiographic view showing thrombosis and sealing of distal guidewire perforation following local injection of thrombin via balloon catheter lumen. No contrast staining is seen.

Shortly thereafter the patient complained of some chest discomfort and it was recognized that there was a distal guidewire-induced coronary perforation (Fig. 10.4). A balloon was immediately advanced to the distal OM and inflated at 0.5 atmospheres: angiography confirmed that this had prevented any further contrast leak. To try to seal the perforation, the balloon was inflated for 25 minutes, combined with IV protamine (70 mg) to reverse the heparin effect. ReoPro was discontinued and platelet transfusions were ordered. Immediate cardiac echocardiography confirmed a small pericardial effusion without signs of tamponade. Right heart catheterization demonstrated mildly elevated right atrial pressure (9 mmHg), a pulmonary artery (PA) pressure of 32/17 mmHg, a pulmonary capillary wedge (PCW) pressure of 13 mmHg and no convincing hemodynamic evidence to suggest cardiac tamponade.

After 25 minutes of balloon inflation, the balloon was deflated. Angiography demonstrated a persistent contrast leak into the pericardial space and the balloon was immediately reinflated at low pressure. After considering cardiac surgery, we came upon a novel idea to seal the perforation. Topical thrombin was obtained from the operating room. This lyophilized powder was mixed with normal saline and dilute Optiray contrast to achieve a thrombin concentration of 50 IU/ml. The coronary guidewire was withdrawn from the balloon catheter, which was still inflated in the distal OM. After careful aspiration of air, 2 ml of the thrombin mixture (100 IU) was slowly injected via the distal balloon catheter lumen in an attempt to thrombose this small tertiary OM branch vessel. The balloon was kept inflated for c. 5 minutes following the thrombin injection. The balloon was deflated and serial angiography over the next 10 minutes demonstrated complete and persistent occlusion of the distal branch with obliteration of the contrast leak (see Fig. 10.5). The patient returned to the ward in a stable condition and was discharged within 48 hours.

45

Discussion

Coronary artery perforation is a relatively uncommon (0.4%), but morbid, complication during coronary interventions. This complication can be particularly difficult to treat in the setting of combined anticoagulant (heparin) and antiplatelet therapy with glycoprotein IIb/IIIa inhibitors. Cardiac tamponade, and occasionally death, may result from this complication, even when it is recognized and treated in a timely fashion.[1]

Coronary perforation due to coronary guidewires accounts for c. 20% of all coronary perforations during catheter-based revascularization, but is more common with the use of hydrophilic-coated wires and in the presence of glycoprotein IIb/IIIa platelet inhibition.[2,3] Prior to the use of glycoprotein IIb/IIIa platelet inhibitors, these guidewire perforations could easily be managed in most cases with conservative measures, including reversal of heparin and prolonged distal balloon inflation.[1,4] However, when glycoprotein IIb/IIIa platelet inhibitors are used, the reversal of these microperforations appears more problematic and may more often result in cardiac tamponade.

A number of creative solutions have been reported to try to deal with the problem of distal coronary perforation. Since the amount of myocardium supplied by these tertiary vessels is rather small, one reasonable approach is to try to thrombose these distal branches to prevent further blood extravasation and tamponade,[5,6] without particular regard to the small amount of myocardial necrosis that might result from this maneuver. In one case report, gelfoam was injected into the distal vessel using an infusion catheter, with successful sealing of the perforation.[5] In a second case, microcoil embolization was used successfully.[6] Anecdotally, other interventionalists have reported the successful sealing of the perforation by injecting organized thrombus, obtained from the patient's own blood, into the distal coronary bed.

Since these cases are relatively rare, few clinicians have extensive experience with managing this complication. The availability and expertise for injection of gelfoam and/or microcoils does not always exist in centers performing PTCA. Therefore, the technique used in this case has some appeal: thrombin can be kept in the catheterization laboratory, and it is very easy to quickly mix and deliver such a solution via the distal lumen of the inflated balloon catheter. We would recommend a thrombin concentration of 50–100 IU/ml, with a delivery of 2–3 ml. In our case, this was effective in promoting rapid and localized thrombosis of the tertiary branch vessel. We would also recommend a 10–20 minute balloon inflation following the thrombin injection in order to ensure good cross-linking of the fibrin clot.

46

Thus, this technique may provide a useful and widely applicable method for dealing with the troublesome complication of guidewire perforation in the setting of glycoprotein IIb/IIIa inhibitors.

References

1. Ajluni SC, Glazier S, Blankenship L et al. Perforation after percutaneous coronary interventions: clinical, angiography therapeutic observations. *Cathet Cardiovasc Diagn* 1994; **32**:206–12.

2. Wong CM, Kwong Mak GY, Chung DT. Distal coronary artery perforation resulting from the use of hydrophilic coated guidewire in tortuous vessels. *Cathet Cardiovasc Diagn* 1998; **44**:93–6.

3. Corcos T, Favereau X, Guerin Y et al. Recanalization of chronic coronary occlusions using a new hydrophilic guidewire. *Cathet Cardiovasc Diagn* 1998; **44**:83–90.

4. Flynn MS, Aguirre FV, Donohue TJ et al. Conservative management of guidewire coronary artery perforation with pericardial effusion during angioplasty for acute inferior myocardial infarction. *Cathet Cardiovasc Diagn* 1993; **29**:285–8.

5. Dixon SR, Webster MW, Ormiston JA et al. Gelfoam embolization of a distal coronary artery guidewire perforation. *Cathet Cardiovasc Intervent* 2000; **49**:214–17.

6. Gaxiola E, Browne KF. Coronary artery perforation repair using microcoil embolization. *Cathet Cardiovasc Diagn* 1998; **43**:474–6.

Case 11

CORONARY RUPTURE AND TAMPONADE

Michael JB Kutryk

Background

This 58-year-old male had presented 1 month previously with new-onset unstable angina/threatened anterolateral myocardial infarction. He was treated with streptokinase, with no rise in creatine kinase (CK) or CKMB fraction. Further symptoms with CCS class IV angina occurred 10 days prior to procedure.

Clinical information

Cardiac risk factors included: current cigarette smoking, a family history of premature coronary disease, hypercholesterolemia and type 2 diabetes mellitus (oral hypoglycemics). The patient did not have hypertension.

Baseline electrocardiogram (ECG): flattened T-waves I, aVL and V3–V6.

Medications at the time of procedure included: ASA, simvastatin, metoprolol, isosorbide mononitrate, gliclazide and metformin.

A diagnostic angiogram showed 80% stenoses of both the left anterior descending (LAD) artery (segment 7) and the first diagonal branch (D1), and a 50% stenosis of the circumflex (Cx) (2 mm vessel).

He was transferred from the referral center for percutaneous transluminal coronary angioplasty (PTCA). The plan was to treat lesions in LAD 7 band D1, and, if symptoms persisted, then the Cx lesion would be treated at a later time.

Angiographic commentary

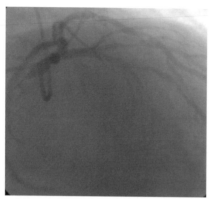

Figure 11.1. *A Judkins left 5, 6 French (Fr) guide catheter was chosen. In this image the 80% lesion can be seen in the LAD (lower vessel) and an 80% lesion in the D1 (upper vessel).*

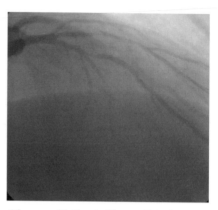

Figure 11.2. *A Choice PT plus guidewire is shown in D1.*

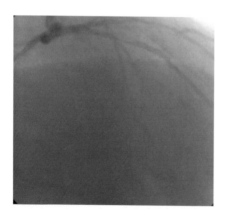

Figure 11.3. *Direct stenting of LAD 7 with a NIR Stent, 3.0 × 32 mm.*

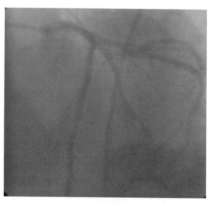

Figure 11.4. *Post-stent implantation in LAD 7. With removal of the balloon, the wire in D1 was inadvertently drawn back into the LAD. The wire was repositioned in the right superior oblique view.*

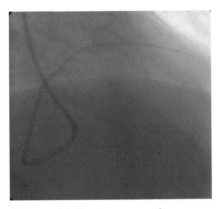

Figure 11.5. *Attempt at direct stenting of D1, using a NIR stent, 3.0 × 32 mm. We were unable to track the stent distally and so the attempt was aborted.*

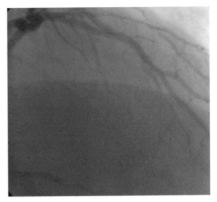

Figure 11.6. *This image was recorded immediately after the attempt at direct stent implantation of D1. Note that the wire is no longer in the main vessel; it was inadvertently repositioned into a side branch of D1. In this angiographic view this went unnoticed.*

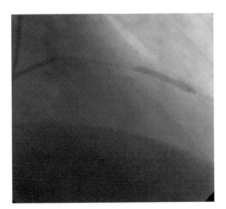

Figure 11.7. *Predilatation PTCA of distal segment of D1.*

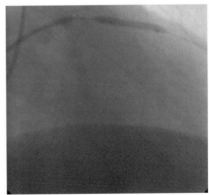

Figure 11.8. *Predilatation PTCA of proximal D1.*

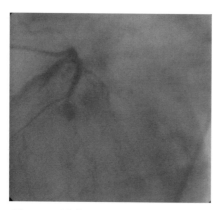

Figure 11.9. Wire repositioned in main D1; pericardial blush observed.

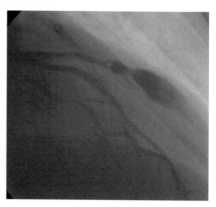

Figure 11.10. Expanding pericardial blush. Patient rapidly decompensated. Precipitous drop in blood pressure with loss of consciousness. Pericardiocentesis performed with placement of pericardial drain. Blood collected for autotransfusion.

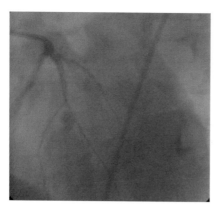

Figure 11.11. Positioning of JoStent polytetrafluoroethylene (PTFE)-covered stent.

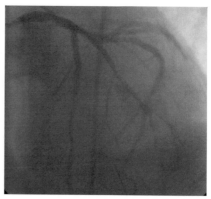

Figure 11.12. Post-JoStent PTFE-covered stent implantation. No extravasation of contrast was seen. Type C dissection noted beyond LAD 7 stent.

52

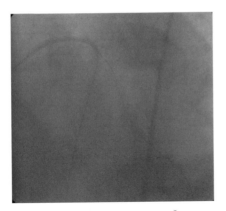

Figure 11.13. *Positioning of stent in LAD 8.*

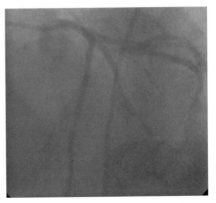

Figure 11.14. *Patient admitted to Coronary Care Unit. Trivial amounts of drainage from pericardial space after stenting procedure. Pericardial drain removed 18 hours post-procedure. Peak CK of 347 IU/l with CKMB of 42 IU/l. Patient was discharged home well 3 days post-procedure.*

Commentary

This case has several important features. First, it underlines the importance of checking wire position in orthogonal views to ensure proper positioning. In this instance, the wire in D1 was placed in a right superior oblique view in which the side branch and main vessel were overlapping.

A life-threatening complication was successfully treated simply and efficiently in this case using a PTFE-covered stent. Remarkably, only a small amount of myocardial damage resulted (peak CK 347 IU/l). This complication could have been avoided with more careful attention to detail.

Case 12

CORONARY RUPTURE AFTER STENTING

Haresh Mehta and Bernhard Meier

Background

Coronary intervention over the years has made rapid strides. With the introduction of better quality hardware and supplementary antiplatelet medications, the procedure is relatively safe with a low incidence of complications. Nevertheless, we present an interesting case of a patient who initially presented with an acute coronary syndrome. The course of events that followed the first intervention, presenting a gamut of complications and sequelae, is noteworthy.

Case report

A 72-year-old male patient presented for the first time with an acute coronary syndrome and the subsequent coronary angiogram demonstrated two-vessel disease (2VD) with complex bifurcation stenoses of the left anterior descending (LAD) coronary artery and the second diagonal branch (D2) (Fig. 12.1), and also a significant lesion in the left circumflex (LCx) coronary artery. The LAD and the D2 were successfully dilated and stented in a 'T' fashion – 3.0 × 18 mm Multilink Stent (ACS) in the LAD and a 2.5 × 8 mm Bestent (Medtronic) in the D2 (Dg; Fig. 12.2). It was decided to dilate the LCx in a second session 3 months later.

Two months later the patient was readmitted with unstable angina and the angiogram showed a tight in-stent restenosis of both the LAD and the D2 (Fig. 12.3). While inflating a 2.5 mm Bonnie balloon (Boston Scientific) within the stent in the D2, the balloon kept slipping back, resulting in a suboptimal result. To circumvent this, the balloon was advanced partially beyond the stent and inflated at 18 atmospheres. The segment of the balloon extending beyond the stent overgrew its predefined diameter and the patient experienced a sharp excruciating pain. Subsequent contrast injection showed a ruptured diagonal branch beyond the stent (Fig. 12.4), with rapid

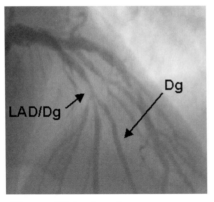

Figure 12.1. Initial angiogram showing the bifurcation stenoses of the LAD and the D2 (LAD/Dg).

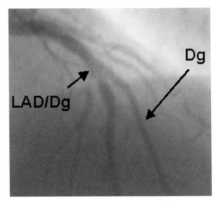

Figure 12.2. Final result after bifurcation stenting of the LAD and the D2 (LAD/Dg).

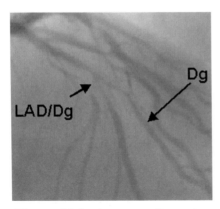

Figure 12.3. Angiogram 2 months later showing restenoses in the stented bifurcation of the LAD and the D2 (LAD/Dg).

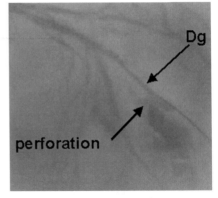

Figure 12.4. Rupture of the diagonal branch (short arrow) into the pericardium.

development of cardiac tamponade. Immediate pericardiocentesis was initiated and the balloon was reinflated in the diagonal branch to temporarily seal the perforation. The blood drained from the pericardium was reinjected into a sheath placed in the femoral vein using a closed system. An attempt was made to seal the perforation with a stent graft [JoMed stent 2.5 × 20 mm, where two stents are mounted one within the other with a polytetrafluoroethylene (PTFE) membrane between them], but this was unsuccessful as the stent could not negotiate down into the diagonal branch and slipped off the balloon onto the wire in the left main stem. All attempts to capture the stent, even with the small profile 1.5 mm Viva balloon (Boston Scientific), proved impossible and hence the stent could not be retrieved back into the guiding catheter. Subsequently, the Viva balloon was partially inflated and used as a plough to push the stent down into the LAD as far as possible. The stent could not be passed beyond the proximal part of the LAD (Fig. 12.5); therefore, it was permanently implanted in that position with repeated inflations of the Viva balloon and the initial 2.5 mm Bonnie balloon. At this moment, the LAD was completely occluded distal to the stent graft (Fig. 12.6) with significant ST elevation in the anterior leads and development of severe angina. The persistently bleeding diagonal branch was now cannulated with a tracker catheter (Target Therapeutics, 0.018 inch diameter), as even the smallest balloon could not be negotiated through the covered stent. Two pieces of a 0.018 inch Cook coil were inserted through the tracker catheter and the perforation was successfully sealed (Fig. 12.6), with loss of the diagonal branch which was devoid of collaterals. The occluded LAD was recanalized (Fig. 12.7) with a Magnum wire (Boston Scientific, 0.014 inch) and the 2.5 mm Bonnie balloon. The chest pain abated and the echocardiogram (ECG) normalized. The pericardial drain was removed the next day and the maximum creatine kinase (CK) was 1500 IU/l, which was attributed to the occluded diagonal branch.

Seven days after the intervention the patient was admitted to the intensive care unit with an acute episode of chest pain and ventricular tachycardia,

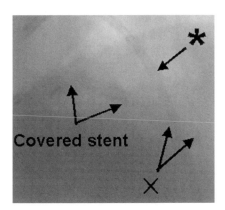

Figure 12.5. Covered stent deployed in the proximal LAD (wide arrows). (*), The pericardiocentesis catheter; (x), the restenosed bifurcation stents.

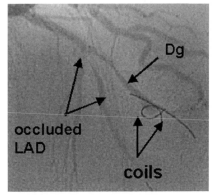

Figure 12.6. Occluded LAD after implantation of the stent graft (wide arrows). Two coils are visible in the ruptured diagonal branch (Dg).

57

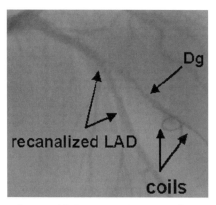

Figure 12.7. *Recanalization of the LAD (long arrows) and sealing of the perforation with coils (small arrows).*

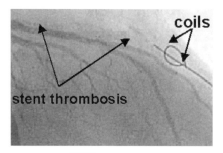

Figure 12.8. *Subacute thrombosis of the covered stent (long arrows) 7 days after placement.*

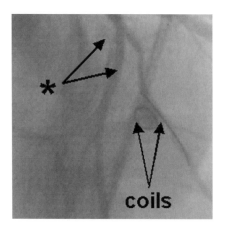

Figure 12.9. *Successful recanalization of the thrombosed LAD (*).*

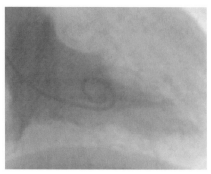

Figure 12.10. *Initial angiogram showing normal LV function with no regional wall motion abnormality.*

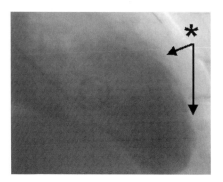

Figure 12.11. *LV angiogram performed after the episode of the first subacute stent thrombosis showing depressed LV function with anteroapical akinesia (*), which is persistent to date.*

58

which was successfully cardioverted, and the ECG showed ST elevations in the anterior leads. The re-angiogram showed a subacute thrombosis of the covered stent (Fig. 12.8), which was successfully recanalized (Fig. 12.9) with a Magnum wire (Boston Scientific) and a 2.5 × 20 mm Magnarail balloon (Boston Scientific). A bolus of abciximab, followed by a 12-hour infusion, was also administered. The diagonal branch was now open but with poor antegrade flow. At this time the LCx stenosis was also dilated and stented. The left ventricular (LV) angiogram, which had been normal during the first intervention (Fig. 12.10), now showed anteroseptal akinesia (Fig. 12.11). The maximum CK was 2647 IU/l. While in the intensive care unit, 3 days after the last intervention, the patient re-experienced another episode of acute chest pain with repeat ST elevation in the anterior leads and the angiogram once again demonstrated a subacute thrombosis of the covered stent, which was again recanalized with a Magnum wire and a Magnarail balloon, under cover of a tirofiban infusion which was continued for 24 hours. The subsequent course was uneventful and the patient was discharged on anti-failure treatment. The ECG now showed Q-waves in the anterior leads.

The patient was readmitted twice after this. On one occasion an in-stent restenosis of the covered stent in the LAD was dilated using a Magnum wire and a 2.5 × 20 mm Adante balloon (Boston Scientific).

The last coronary angiogram, 6 months after the last intervention, did not reveal any restenosis but the LV function was still depressed [ejection fraction (EF) 45%], with persistent anteroapical akinesia. The patient was discharged with the recommendation to attend a cardiac rehabilitation program. He has remained free of symptoms for 1 year since.

Discussion

The case presented above is an excellent example of complications seldom encountered and also presents different methods that can be employed to overcome them. Coronary artery ruptures, although rare, can be fatal if not expeditiously managed. Many methods have been described for handling such complications. One of these is the use of covered stents[1,2] to seal the perforations, which in this case was unsuccessful due to difficulty in negotiating down to the perforation. Difficulty to negotiate has been seen mainly in calcified and tortuous vessels, as these stents are bulkier than uncovered stents. This could be a limitation of covered stents as calcified vessels are more prone to rupture. Other methods that have been described include injection of precoagulated autologous blood[3] and embolization of

59

coils,[4,5] which was successfully employed in this case. These two methods can be pursued if the area at risk is not too large and can be sacrificed. All of these measures obviate the need for an emergency coronary artery bypass graft (CABG), with its associated morbidity and increased mortality in emergency situations.

Various coated stents have been employed (autologous veins, PTFE, etc.) to seal perforations and to reduce distal embolizations,[6] especially in degenerated venous grafts. Coated stents have also been described in reports to reduce restenosis,[7] stent thrombosis and target vessel revascularization[8] rates, which ironically occurred repeatedly in this case, resulting in re-infarcts and depressed left ventricular function, thereby raising the question of whether covered stents really reduce restenosis and stent thrombosis or act as a nidus for the same. A report by Campbell et al[9] demonstrated two cases of covered stents, one of which developed subacute stent thrombosis at 1 month, and another which developed proliferative and occlusive restenosis. An aggressive and prolonged medication might help to prevent these complications in covered stents. This issue needs to be addressed in randomized trials.

Regarding this case, the question arises of whether CABG would have been a better treatment option. However, with this coronary anatomy both options seemed reasonable and the patient's preference was honored.

References

1. Caputo RP, Amin N, Marvasti M et al. Successful treatment of a saphenous vein graft perforation with an autologous vein-covered stent. *Cathet Cardiovasc Intervent* 1999; **48**:382–6.

2. Ramsdale Dr, Mushahwar SS, Morris JL. Repair of coronary artery perforation after rotastenting by implantation of the JoStent covered stent. *Cathet Cardiovasc Diagn* 1998; **45**:310–13.

3. Hadjimiltiades S, Paraskevaides S, Kazinakis G, Louridas G. Coronary vessel perforation during balloon angioplasty: a case report. *Cathet Cardiovasc Diagn* 1998; **45**:417–20.

4. Gaxiola E, Browne KF. Coronary artery perforation repair using microcoil embolization. *Cathet Cardiovasc Diagn* 1998; **43**:474–6.

5. Dorros G, Jain A, Kumar K. Management of coronary artery rupture: covered stent or microcoil embolization. *Cathet Cardiovasc Diagn* 1995; **36**:148–54.

6. Briguori C, De Gregorio J, Nishida T et al. Polytetrafluoroethylene-covered stent for the treatment of narrowings in aorticocoronary saphenous vein grafts. *Am J Cardiol* 2000; **86**:343–6.

7. Baldus S, Koster R, Reimers J, Hamm CW. Membrane-covered stents for the treatment of aortocoronary vein graft disease. *Cathet Cardiovasc Intervent* 2000; **50**:83–8.

8. Stefanadis C, Toutouzas K, Tsiamis E et al. Stents covered by autologous venous grafts: feasibility and immediate and long-term results. *Am Heart J* 2000; **139**:437–45.

9. Campbell PG, Hall JA, Harcombe AA, de Belder MA. The Jomed covered stent graft for coronary artery aneurysms and acute perforation: a successful device which needs careful deployment and may not reduce restenosis. *J Invasive Cardiol* 2000; **12**:272–6.

Case 13

UNPREDICTABILITY OF SIMPLE PERCUTANEOUS CORONARY INTERVENTION (PCI)

Kostantinos S Spargias and Ian M Penn

Background

A 62-year-old woman was admitted to hospital with the diagnosis of acute coronary syndrome. Her 12-lead echocardiogram (ECG) exhibited progressive T-wave inversion in the anterior leads and her troponin was elevated. She was therefore referred for coronary angiography, which she underwent on day 3 of hospitalization. She had first presented with unstable angina symptoms 5 years before and she underwent circumflex (Cx) percutaneous transluminal coronary angioplasty (PTCA) at that time. A 50% stenosis in the mid-left anterior descending (LAD) coronary artery was noted then. Her other past medical history was unremarkable.

Angiographic commentary

Coronary angiography revealed a disease-free left main stem, maintained patency result of the previous Cx PTCA and mild irregularities in the right coronary artery (RCA). However, the previously described moderate LAD disease had progressed to a rather long (c. 23 mm) and severely stenotic (c. 90%) lesion, initiating at the origin of the second diagonal branch (D2) (Fig. 13.1). Left ventricular (LV) angiography demonstrated severe anteroapical hypokinesis. As the indication for revascularization was clear, we proceeded to *ad hoc* LAD PCI.

Discussion

At first glance there is nothing outstanding in this case, an unexceptional

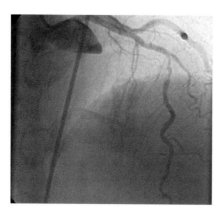

Figure 13.1. Long mid-LAD lesion.

Monday morning procedure. However, the 'unexpected' complication that ensued during the PCI makes it a case worth reporting and discussing.

It was quite clear that the previously described moderate LAD lesion had progressed to a significant stenosis. The pace of this progression was difficult to surmise. However, both the severe anterior wall hypokinesis and the myocardial enzyme release attested to a recent, temporary occlusive lesion. Furthermore, the lack of anginal symptoms up to the current admission supports the argument that a recent rupture within the plaque probably resulted in an acute rise in the stenosis grade. On QCA, the reference LAD diameter was *c.* 3.0 mm and angiographically the lesion was not calcified. A 'soft' lesion would be expected to be suitable for primary stenting.

In view of all of the above, our strategy was to predilate the lesion with a 2.5 mm diameter balloon and then cover it using a 3.0 mm diameter stent.

The diagonal branch emanating from the proximal margin of the lesion was not of concern, since it was a rather small artery (≤1.5 mm) and its origin was relatively disease-free. Therefore, no plans were made to intervene in or to protect this branch.

The initial predilatation with a 2.5 mm diameter compliant balloon (Viva Primo, Boston Scientific) at 14 atmospheres resulted in a dog-bone-like picture and reduced the maximum stenosis from *c.* 90 to <50% (Fig. 13.2a and b). Additional dilatation was not performed, as the balloon used was considered undersized for this purpose. It was also felt that the residual stenosis would not hamper appropriate stent expansion and further predilatation with a larger balloon was not performed for logistic reasons. However, the section with the residual stenosis proved to be resilient even to the larger 3.0 mm diameter stent-deploying balloon (3.0 × 28 mm BioDivysio, BioCompatibles) inflated up to 16 atmospheres (Fig. 13.3a and b). At that point, a decision was made to use a short 3.5 mm compliant balloon (3.5 × 10 mm Cross Sail, Guidant), rendering a *c.* 1:2:1 balloon to

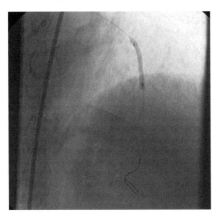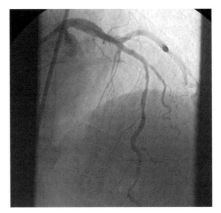

Figure 13.2a and b. *The mid-LAD lesion is predilated with a 2.5 × 20 mm Viva Primo balloon at 16 atmospheres (Boston Scientific). Note that due to balloon underexpansion and acute vessel-wall recoil there is c. 50% residual stenosis after predilatation.*

artery ratio, for postdilatation of the hard undilatable in-stent section. Still, the plaque remained rigid and undilatable at 16 atmospheres, with the balloon resuming a more manifest dog-bone configuration (Fig. 13.4). This resulted in a perforation at the level of the distal part of the balloon with free and brisk contrast extravasation into the pericardium (Fig. 13.5).

The perforation was successfully sealed with a coronary stent graft [polytetrafluoroethylene (PTFE)-covered JoStent, JoMed] (Fig. 13.6a and b). The ischemic time (balloon inflation causing perforation to sealing inflation with stent graft) was 5 minutes, and could have been even shorter had a premounted graft stent been available in our laboratory.

Commentary

Coronary artery perforation is a rare but life-threatening complication of PCI. Its incidence varies according to the devices used and it is estimated to be 0.1–0.2% with conventional PTCA, and substantially higher incidences of up to 3% have been reported with the so-called debulking devices.[1] The incidence of this complication has increased with the aggressive use of oversized balloons and stents, and higher pressures, to optimize the acute stent cross-sectional area (CSA), complicating c. 1% of stent procedures.[2–6] Other identifiable causes of coronary perforation are balloon rupture (at high inflation pressures and/or within calcific segments), aggressive debulking with

65

directional coronary atherectomy (DCA), rotational atherectomy or excimer laser coronary atherectomy (ELCA) and guidewire perforation.[2,6,7] Features associated with perforation include balloon to artery ratios of 1:2:1 [on QCA or intravascular ultrasound (IVUS)] or more, complex lesion morphology, small vessel diameter, heavy calcification and use of a compliant balloon.[2,6,7]

In retrospect, use of a 3.0 mm non-compliant balloon might have been a more appropriate option. This would have resulted in a balloon to artery ratio of <1:1:1 and more a equally distributed stretching force would have

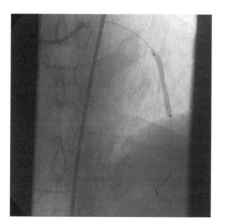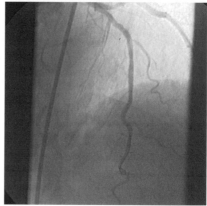

Figure 13.3a and b. *A 3.0 × 28 mm BioDivysio stent is deployed at 16 atmospheres. Note the dog-bone-like configuration and the residual stenosis due to incomplete stent expansion.*

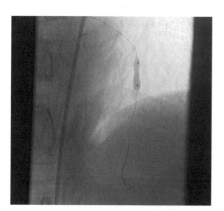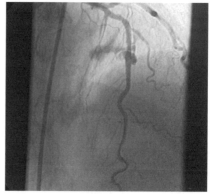

Figure 13.4. *The stent is postdilated using a compliant 3.5 × 10 mm Cross Sail balloon (Guidant) at 16 atmospheres. Note the marked dog-bone configuration of the balloon.*

Figure 13.5. *Perforation of the LAD and free contrast extravasation into the pericardium at the point of the distal overexpansion of the postdilatation balloon.*

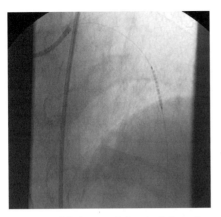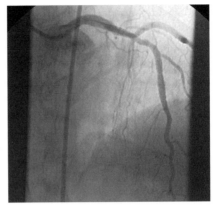

Figure 13.6a and b. *A 3.5 × 9 mm PTFE-covered JoStent (JoMed) is deployed at the site of the perforation, successfully sealing it.*

been applied along the entire length of the balloon, making the 'dog-bone' configuration less likely to occur.

Some localized perforations can be managed with prolonged (perfusion) balloon inflation and reversal of heparin with protamine.[2,3] Urgent echocardiography is mandatory in this complication and, together with clinical symptoms and signs, will diagnose frank or threatened tamponade, determining the need for pericardiocentesis.[2,3] In our case, the total 'extravasation time' through the perforation was <1 minute and the ECG showed a tiny rim of pericardial fluid.

There are anecdotal reports of the successful seal of coronary perforation following conventional balloon angioplasty with the use of a common stent. It appears that the success of this approach depends on the course and direction of the perforating tear in the artery wall, and it may often leave the perforation unaffected or even aggravate it.

Until recently, if the above approaches failed then urgent surgery was mandatory and was necessary in up to 50% of perforations. Coronary perforation carried a high mortality (15–30%) and morbidity, acute myocardial infarction (AMI) in 30–40%.[2,5]

More recently, there have been some developments with important ramifications for the management of a coronary perforation. First, the advent of PTFE-covered stents allowed for a definitive percutaneous treatment of acute perforation while maintaining vessel patency.[1,8,9] Distal perforations in small coronary arteries and the presence of severe tortuosity proximal to the perforation are limitations of this new treatment modality. According to recent reports, this approach can reduce the mortality of coronary perforation to <10%.[8,9]

The increasing use of glycoprotein IIb/IIIa platelet receptor inhibitors, as pharmacological adjuvants to PCI, would be very relevant in the event of coronary perforation. The potential for more prolonged or even delayed bleeding into the pericardium is genuine when these agents are used. In addition, while heparin is readily reversed with protamine, reversal of the chimeric monoclonal antibody-type inhibitor (abciximax) requires time-consuming platelet transfusions, while there is no currently available means of reversing the action of small molecule inhibitors (eptifibatide and tirofiban). Of course, the latter are short-acting agents and their antiplatelet effects wane within 3–4 hours. No glycoprotein IIa/IIIb inhibitor had been used in our patient, making these considerations irrelevant in this particular case.

References

1. Elsner M, Zeiher AM. Perforation and rupture of coronary arteries. *Herz* 1998; **23**:311–18.

2. Kutryk MJB, Serruys PV. *Coronary Stenting. Current Perspectives.* 1st edn. (Martin Dunitz Ltd: London, 1999) 252–3.

3. Colombo A, Tobis J. *Techniques in Coronary Artery Stenting*, 1st edn. (Martin Dunitz Ltd: London, 2000) 265–8.

3. Alfonso F, Goicolea A, Gaglione A et al. Arterial perforation during optimization of coronary stents using high-pressure balloon inflations. *Am J Cardiol* 1996; **78**:1169–72.

5. Hall P. Nakamura S, Maiello L et al. Factors associated with procedural complications during high pressure optimized Palmaz–Schatz intracoronary stent implantation. *Circulation* 1994; **90**:I612.

6. Benzuly KH, Glazier S, Grines CL et al. Coronary perforation: an unreported complication after intracoronary stent implantation. *J Am Coll Cardiol* 1996; **27**:253A.

7. Reimers B, von Birgelen C, van der Giessen WJ, Serruys PW. A word of caution on optimizing stent deployment in calcified lesion: acute coronary rupture with cardiac tamponade. *Am Heart J* 1996; **131**:192–4.

8. Briguori C, Anzuini A, Corvaja N et al. Emergency PTFE-covered stent implantation to treat coronary ruptures. *Circulation* 2000; **102**:I640.

9. Briguori C, Nishida T, Anzuini A et al. Emergency polytetrafluoroethylene-covered stent implantation to treat coronary ruptures. *Circulation* 2000; **102**:3028–31.

Case 14

Extraction Of Large Intracoronary Thrombus In Acute Myocardial Infarction (AMI) By Percutaneous Fogarty Maneuver – Intentional 'Abuse' Of A Novel Interventional Device

Dietrich Baumgart, Holger Eggebrecht, Christoph K Naber, Olaf Dirsch, Michael Haude and Raimund Erbel

Background

Intracoronary thrombus in the infarct-related artery (IRA) remains a challenge for interventional catheter-based techniques in AMI and may result in severe complications due to distal embolization. We describe a patient with AMI in whom a large intracoronary thrombus of the left anterior descending (LAD) coronary artery was successfully removed by a percutaneous 'Fogarty maneuver' using an expanded filter protection device.

Introduction

Intracoronary thrombus in the IRA remains a challenge for interventional catheter-based techniques in AMI. Downstream embolization of thrombotic material during balloon inflation or stent deployment results in deterioration of distal flow, loss of side branches and further infarct extension.[1,2] Besides fibrinolytic and thrombolytic agents,[3,4] catheter aspiration,[5] thrombectomy devices (X-sizer, AngioJet, TEC),[6–8] ultrasound thrombolysis[9] and, more recently, distal protection devices[1] have all been used to mechanically reduce clot burden and the risk of embolization.

69

In the present report we describe a patient with AMI in whom a large intracoronary thrombus was removed from the coronary circulation by a percutaneous Fogarty maneuver using an expanded filter protection device.

Case report

A 32-year-old male patient with no prior history of cardiac disease presented 4 hours from onset of symptoms with evolving anteroapical myocardial infarction.

Cardiovascular risk factors included current smoking, hypercholesterolemia and obesity. Due to chronic migraine headache, the patient was treated with verapamil, prednisone and sumatriptan, the latter of which is known to increase thrombogenicity as well as vasoconstriction.

The 12-lead electrocardiogram (ECG) showed ST-segment elevations in leads V4–V6, as well as in I, II and AVF (Fig. 14.1). The initial creatine kinase (CK) concentration was normal at 62 IU/l, troponin I was slightly elevated (0.2 ng/ml) and the initial myoglobin was elevated at 158 IU/l.

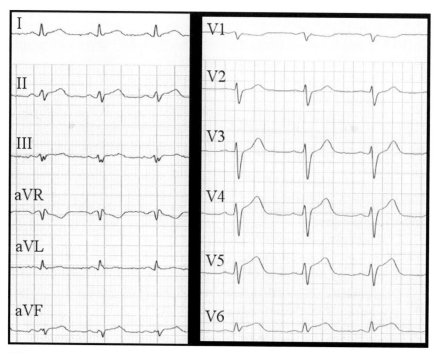

Figure 14.1. *Twelve-lead ECG at presentation showing ST-segment elevations in leads V4–V6, as well as in I, II and AVF.*

Immediate selective injection of the left coronary artery (LCA) showed a large filling defect in the proximal LAD coronary artery, arousing suspicions of intracoronary thrombus formation (Fig. 14.2). The distal LAD was occluded, presumably due to thrombotic embolization. The left circumflex (LCx) artery showed an anomalous uptake from the right coronary artery (RCA), both without angiographic evidence of flow-limiting coronary artery disease.

Intravascular ultrasound (IVUS) was performed to further evaluate the nature of the filling defect. IVUS showed a low reflecting structure with a typical layering which almost occluded the lumen, confirming the suspicion of intracoronary thrombus formation (Stary class VIb;[10] Fig. 14.2). Proximal and distal to the lesion, only discrete atherosclerotic wall alterations (Stary class III[10]) were noted.

At the beginning of the intervention, a weight-adapted bolus of the glycoprotein IIb/IIIa receptor inhibitor abciximab (0.25 mg/kg body weight; ReoPro, Centocor Lilly, Indianapolis, IN) was administered IV and a continuous 12-hour infusion of 10 µg/min was commenced to prevent an apposition thrombus in the vessel. The LAD was intubated with an 8 French (Fr) Judkins left guiding catheter (Supertorque Plus; Cordis, Warren, NJ), and 10 000 IU of heparin were administered intraarterially. A 0.014 inch guidewire (Hi-Torque Floppy II; ACS, Santa Clara, CA) was placed into the distal LAD after uneventful crossing of the lesion.

Based on IVUS findings showing a large thrombus burden and rather discrete coronary atherosclerosis, an attempt was made to mechanically extract the thrombus burden, as pharmacologic dissolution was not observed macroscopically.

To prevent further downstream embolization during consecutive catheter manipulation, a 6.0 mm filter protection device (AngioGuard; Cordis, Warren, NJ) was placed into the distal LAD. The filter device is a standard 0.014 inch guidewire which contains a self-expanding nitinol basket with a

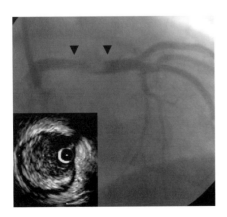

Figure 14.2. *Initial angiogram of the LCA showing a large filling defect (arrow heads) in the proximal segment of the LAD. VUS showing a low reflecting structure with a typical layering which almost occluded the lumen (Stary class VIb).*

71

polyurethane porous membrane at the distal wire end. The filter pores measure 100 μm, which allows distal perfusion during the filtering process. The basket is preloaded in a delivery sheath and after crossing the lesion the filter is deployed by withdrawal of the delivery sheath. With the expanded filter preventing distal embolization of atherothrombotic material, coronary angioplasty and/or stent placement is performed. Then, the filter is retrieved by the use of a capture sheath, and the collapsed filter and capture sheath can be retracted.

In a first attempt, a 5 Fr monorail aspiration catheter (Export; PercuSurge/Medtronic) was advanced to the lesion and repeat manual suction of a total of 30 ml of blood was applied. Filtering of the aspirate, however, showed only discrete thrombotic particles with no luminal enlargement or reduction of the filling defect by angiography.

Therefore, we decided to withdraw the expanded filter protection device from the distal LAD up to the retrieval sheath, placed in the ostium of the LAD, to retrieve the large residual thrombus by a Fogarty maneuver (Fig. 14.3). To prevent possible systemic embolization, the guiding catheter was deeply seated in the LAD ostium without obstructing inflow or damping of pressure.

After first withdrawal over the lesion, a thrombus particle of *c.* 2 × 2 mm was found in the filter basket. The Fogarty maneuver was repeated three times. Post-interventional angiography showed significant reduction of the filling defect with almost no residual luminal obstruction (Fig. 14.4). IVUS confirmed the angiographic findings as it showed a wall-adherent, echodense residual thrombus with significant reduction of the thrombus burden (Fig.14.4).

Recanalization of the distal LAD occlusion was attempted using balloon angioplasty. However, flow could not be re-established by repeat mechanical fragmentation and dilatation with a 2.5/20 mm balloon catheter (Europass; Cordis, Warren, NJ).

Post-interventional course showed a maximal rise of CK to 1118 IU/l; the maximal troponin I concentration was 65.6 ng/ml. The patient developed a

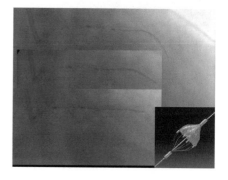

Figure 14.3. *Retraction of the expanded filter device through the proximal LAD to mechanically extract clot using a Fogarty maneuver.*

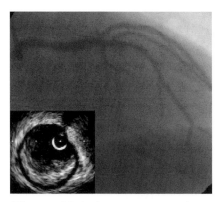

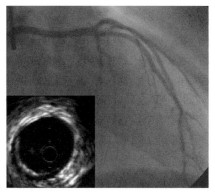

Figure 14.4. *Post-interventional angiography showing significant reduction of the proximal filling defect with almost no residual luminal obstruction. IVUS showed wall-adherent, echodense residual thrombus with significant reduction of the thrombus burden.*

Figure 14.5. *Six-month follow-up angiography showing a good long-term result of the proximal lesion with spontaneously recanalized distal LAD. IVUS revealed a healed, wall-adherent remnant of the former thrombus.*

left ventricular (LV) anteroapical aneurysm with thrombus formation and was therefore anticoagulated with phenprocoumon. Six-month follow-up angiography showed a good long-term result of the proximal lesion with spontaneously recanalized distal LAD (Fig. 14.5). IVUS revealed a wall-adherent consolidation with a healed, eccentric remnant of the former thrombus (Fig. 14.5). The ventriculography showed an apical aneurysm with moderate reduction of systolic LV function (Fig. 14.6).

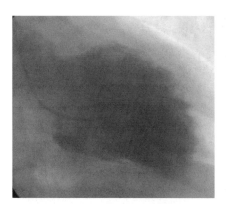

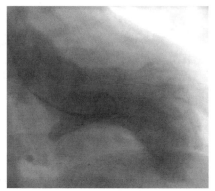

Figure 14.6. *Ventriculography showing a large anteroapical ventricular aneurysm (left – diastole, right – systole).*

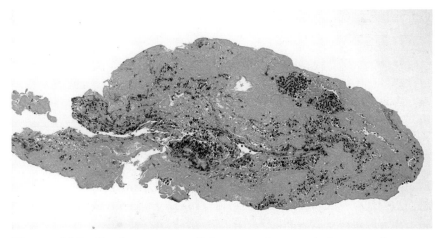

Figure 14.7. *Histologic picture of the retrieved material showing a large, fresh thrombus particle (100X, H&E).*

For pathologic analysis of the material captured within the filter, the filter basket was fixed in 4% buffered formalin. Small particles were retrieved with a fine forceps and paraffin embedding was performed following standard techniques. Sections of 4 μm were cut and stained with hematoxylin eosin (H&E). The rest of the material was processed on slides using a cytocentrifuge; the slides were also H&E stained.

Histologic examination showed a large particle of fresh thrombus material without evidence of vessel wall structures or atherosclerotic material (Fig. 14.7).

Discussion

Disruption of atherosclerotic plaques and intracoronary thrombus formation is widely accepted as the main pathophysiological cause for the development of acute coronary syndromes.[11] IV thrombolysis and percutaneous transluminal coronary angioplasty (PTCA) are well established reperfusion therapies for AMI. Besides increased bleeding complications, thrombolysis has been reported to be unsuccessful in recanalizing the occluded artery in c. 20% of patients.[12] Previous investigators found primary PTCA of the culprit lesion to be superior to thrombolysis in AMI.[13] The presence of intracoronary thrombus has been identified as a predictor of unfavorable results because of distal embolization of no-reflow phenomenon.[7,14]

Several catheter-based approaches have been introduced to mechanically reduce clot burden prior to angioplasty and thereby reduce the risk of embolization.[6,9] Also, pharmacologic dissolution of pre-existing intracoronary thrombus has been reported after administration of glycoprotein IIb/IIIa receptor inhibitors.[15] With the advent of distal protection devices (e.g. Percusurge Guardwire, AngioGuard filter device), a new alternative for prevention of downstream embolization during angioplasty is available.[1]

The present case is unique in several ways. First, intracoronary thrombosis was presumably related to sumatriptan medication because of the presence of minimal discrete coronary atherosclerotic plaques, as this has been previously described as a not infrequent side effect of this drug.[16,17] Also, prednisone is known to increase thrombogenicity. Despite the presence of cardiovascular risk factors, IVUS could not demonstrate either plaque rupture nor significant coronary atherosclerosis. Therefore, we decided to mechanically reduce clot burden rather than obviating stent placement with the inherent risk for restenosis in a young patient. Additionally, the glycoprotein IIb/IIIa inhibitor abciximab was administered to stop further appositional thrombus formation.

We initially intended to use catheter aspiration to reduce clot burden. However, manual suction with a dedicated aspiration catheter was found to be ineffective.

This patient had an anomalous origin of the LCx from the RCA, there being no major side branches proximal to the LAD lesion. We therefore decided to retract the expanded filter protection device to actively retrieve the thrombus by a Fogarty maneuver. The device used is designed to be placed distal to a stenosis and to passively prevent distal embolization during balloon angioplasty by accumulation of debris in the filter. After the intervention, the filter is designed to be retrieved by a capture sheath. Retraction of the expanded filter basket within the coronary artery during the procedure should normally be prevented, as recommended by the manufacturer, because of the theoretical risk of dissection. However, we found the nitinol basket to be atraumatic to the coronary vessel wall when intentionally retracted during this interventional procedure. (The design of the filter system can be appreciated in the insert in Fig. 14.3.). Whilst the device is described as 'umbrella like' this is actually not the case. An umbrella has potentially sharp and damaging ends to the metal spines that run radially from the center to support the fabric of the umbrella when it is open (expanded). The AngioGuard device does not have these potentially damaging 'spines' that terminate at the edge of the fabric, the 'spines' actually continue to rejoin the body of the device, so presenting an atraumatic curve to the vessel wall.

75

The possibility of drawing thrombus out of the coronary vessel or vein graft, retrograde, into the systemic circulation must be carefully avoided. Thrombus within a vessel will normally only embolize downstream. However, with intentional (or accidental) physical removal of the clot in this way there must be a possibility of 'dropping' it into the systemic circulation where it may then embolize to the cerebral or other important vascular beds. To obviate this possibility, care was taken to maintain engagement of the guiding catheter with the vessel at the time of withdrawal of the thrombus-filled device. Also, the guiding catheter was not flushed until all possible thrombotic material was aspirated.

An important observation from the present case is that distal thrombotic embolization is difficult to manage once it has occurred. This underlines the importance of distal protection devices in situations with large thrombus burdens.

Limitations

We describe successful removal of an intracoronary thrombus by 'abusing' an expanded distal protection device by using it to perform a Fogarty maneuver in a patient with favorable coronary anatomy. The potential risk of coronary artery dissection and systemic embolism is particularly emphasized.

References

1. Belli G, Pezzano A, De Biase AM et al. Adjunctive thrombus aspiration and mechanical protection from distal embolization in primary percutaneous intervention for acute myocardial infarction. *Cathet Cardiovasc Intervent* 2000; **50**:362–70.

2. Saber RS, Edwards WD, Bailey KR. Coronary embolization after balloon angioplasty or thrombolytic therapy: an autopsy study of 32 cases. *J Am Coll Cardiol* 1993; **22**:1283–8.

3 Denardo SJ, Morris NB, Rocha-Singh KJ et al. Safety and efficacy of extended urokinase infusion plus stent deployment for treatment of obstructed, older saphenous vein grafts. *Am J Cardiol* 1995; **76**:776–80.

4. Haude M, Altmann C, Eick B et al. Analysis of vessel wall morphology, blood flow velocity, and the hemostatic system in a patient with a large intracoronary thrombus. *Cathet Cardiovasc Diagn* 1998; **43**:298–305.

5. Murakami T, Mizuno S, Takahashi Y et al. Intracoronary aspiration thrombectomy for acute myocardial infarction. *Am J Cardiol* 1998; **82**:839–44.

6. Ischinger T, X-SIZER Study Group. Thrombectomy with the X-SIZER catheter system in the coronary circulation: initial results from a multi-center study. *J Invasive Cardiol* 2001; **13**:81–8.

7. Nakagawa Y, Matsuo S, Kimura T et al. Thrombectomy with AngioJet catheter in native coronary arteries for patients with acute or recent myocardial infarction. *Am J Cardiol* 1999; **83**:994–9.

8. Topaz O, Bernardo N, Desai P, Janin Y. Acute thrombotic–ischemic coronary syndromes: usefulness of TEC. *Cathet Cardiovasc Intervent* 1999; **48**:406–20.

9. Rosenschein U, Gaul G, Erbel R et al. Percutaneous transluminal therapy of occluded saphenous vein grafts: can the challenge be met with ultrasound thrombolysis? *Circulation* 1999; **99**:26–9.

10. Erbel R, Ge J, Gorge G et al. Intravascular ultrasound classification of atherosclerotic lesions according to American Heart Association recommendation. *Coron Artery Dis* 1999; **10**:489–99.

11. Fuster V, Badimon L, Badimon JJ, Cheesebro JH. The pathogenesis of coronary artery disease and the acute coronary syndromes. *N Engl J Med* 1992; **326**:242–50.

12. The GUSTO Angiographic Investigators. The effects of tissue plasminogen activator, streptokinase, or both on coronary artery patency, ventricular function, and survival after acute myocardial infarction. *N Engl J Med* 1993; **329**:1615–22.

13. Grines CL, Browne KF, Marco et al, for the Primary Angioplasty in Myocardial Infarction Study Group. A comparison of immediate angioplasty with thrombolytic therapy for acute myocardial infarction. *N Engl J Med* 1993; **328**:673–9.

14. Ellis SG, Roubin GS, King SB et al. Angiographic and clinical predictors of acute closure after native vessel coronary angioplasty. *Circulation* 1988; **77**:372–9.

15. Eick B, Haude M, Altmann C et al. Treatment of a large intracoronary thrombus with urokinase and a chimeric monoclonal platelet aggregation inhibitor. *Dtsch Med Wochenschr* 1997; **122**:709–15.

16. Meuller L, Gallagher RM, Ciervo CA. Vasospasm-induced myocardial infarction with sumatriptan. *Headache* 1996; **36**:329–31.

17. Ottervanger JP, Valkenburg HA, Grobbee DE, Stricker BH. Characteristics and determinants of sumatriptan-associated chest pain. *Arch Neurol* 1997; **54**:1387–92.

77

Case 15

SUBACUTE THROMBOTIC OCCLUSION TREATED BY THROMBOSUCTION AND STENTING

Winston Martin and Edoardo Camenzind

Background

A 65-year-old male with type 2 diabetes mellitus and treated hypertension was admitted to our centre with a 2 day history of retrosternal chest pain. An electrocardiogram (ECG) and cardiac enzyme values were consistent with a recent transmural inferoposterior myocardial infarction [admission creatine kinase (CK) 3927 IU/l (normal range 47–222 IU/l), CK myocardial band (MB) activity 330 IU/l (normal range 2–14 IU/l)].

Angiographic commentary

The diagnostic angiogram revealed a complete occlusion of the mid-right coronary artery (RCA) just after the acute marginal branch (Figs. 15.1a and b).

A 7 French (Fr) Vector Judkins right 4.5 guiding catheter (Medtronic) was engaged in the RCA ostium and a 0.014 inch × 190 cm Magnum coronary guidewire (Boston Scientific Scimed) was introduced, but could not traverse the occlusion (Fig. 15.2).

A 0.014 inch × 190 cm PT Graphix guidewire (Boston Scientific Scimed) was advanced through the occlusion with support from a Viva Primo 2.5 × 13 mm angioplasty balloon (Boston Scientific Scimed), which was dottered through the beginning of the occlusion and inflated at 8 atmospheres for 20 seconds (Fig. 15.3).

There was no improvement with failure of flow restoration (Fig. 15.4). A RESCUE aspiration thrombectomy device (Boston Scientific Scimed) was introduced initially up to the start of segment 3 of the RCA (Fig. 15.5), resulting in some flow restoration (TIMI grade 1 flow) with a faint image of the retroventricular branch (Fig. 15.6).

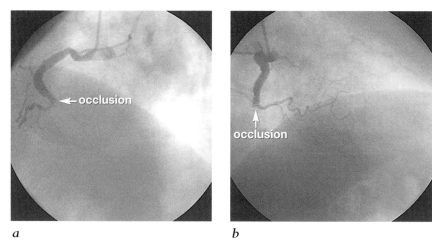

Figure 15.1. (**a**) The diagnostic angiogram in the left anterior oblique (LAO) projection (LAO = 60°) shows that the RCA is occluded just after the acute marginal branch. (**b**) The right anterior oblique projection (RAO = 30°).

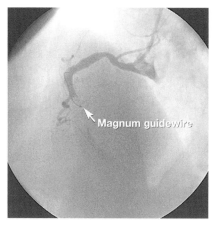 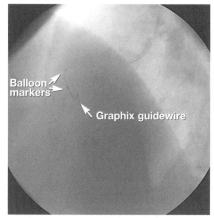

Figure 15.2. Using a 7 Fr Judkins right 4.5 guiding catheter, a Magnum guidewire was unable to cross the occlusion. (LAO = 46°; cranial = 18°).

Figure 15.3. Using balloon support, a Graphix wire was successfully passed through the thrombus into the distal vessel.

After the guidewire was repositioned more distally in the retroventricular branch (Fig. 15.7), two further passes of the RESCUE device extending into the distal artery resulted in significantly improved flow (TIMI grade 2 flow). A number of distal vessel filling defects, indicative of residual thrombus (Fig. 15.8a), could still be seen, despite successful thrombosuction (Fig. 15.9).

80

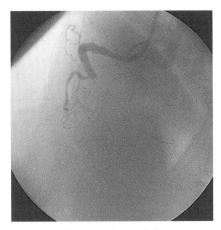

Figure 15.4. *Failure of flow restoration (TIMI grade 0 flow) after dilatation with a 2.5 × 13 mm angioplasty balloon.*

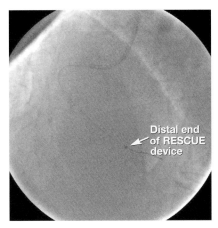

Figure 15.5. *The aspiration thrombectomy device is shown in segment 3 of the vessel.*

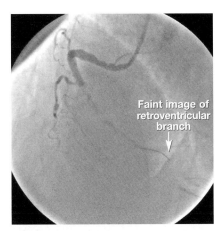

Figure 15.6. *After the initial pass of the aspiration device, TIMI grade 1 flow is now present, with a faint image of the retroventricular branch.*

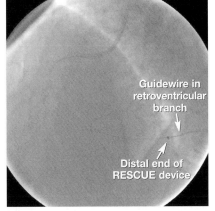

Figure 15.7. *After repositioning of the guidewire in the retroventricular branch, the third pass of the thrombosuction catheter is shown extending further along the distal RCA vessel.*

A significant stenosis was now apparent in segment 2 at the position of the previous occlusion (Figs. 15.8a and b), which was stented using a S670 4.0 × 15 mm stent (Medtronic AVE), giving a good angiographic result with restored TIMI grade 3 flow (Fig. 15.10).

81

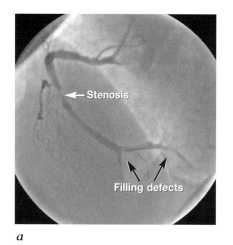

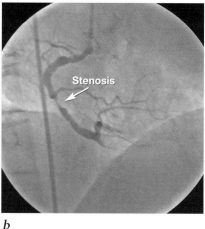

a   *b*

Figure 15.8. *(a) LAO cranial projection and **(b)** RAO projection (RAO =
30°). There is a significant stenosis present at the position of the previous
occlusion with some distal vessel-filling defect abnormalities.*

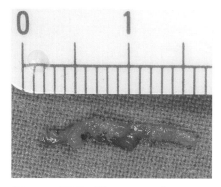

Figure 15.9. *The aspirated
thrombus.*

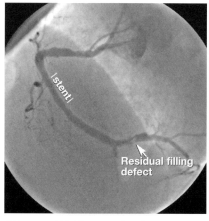

Figure 15.10. *Result after stenting
with a Medtronic AVE S670 4.0 ×
15 mm stent. TIMI grade 3 flow is
restored but filling defects in the
distal vessel and branches persist,
indicating small amounts of residual
thrombus (LAO cranial projection).*

The patient commenced treatment with abciximab (ReoPro; Eli Lilly) and oral clopidogrel Plavix; Sanofi-Synthelabo). The patient underwent a check angiography the following morning which demonstrated a patent vessel with some persistence of thrombus in the distal vessel.

Discussion

This case illustrates some of the difficulties which can be encountered in performing intervention on a subacute thrombotic occlusion.[1] In the immediate acute phase of a myocardial infarction, the restoration of some arterial flow by dispersal of fresh thrombus can be achieved with minimal difficulty, often with the guidewire alone. However, as the thrombus ages over a period of hours it becomes more gelatinous in consistency, making it more difficult to pass through a guidewire and refractory to balloon inflation because of immediate jelly-like recoil. As described here, aspiration thrombectomy may aid intervention on thrombotic occlusions >24 hours old.

The RESCUE thrombosuction catheter is a flexible Monorail catheter which requires a 7 Fr guiding catheter. This is one of the reasons we prefer to use 7 Fr sheaths and catheters for all our acute angioplasties. It is introduced over a prepositioned 0.014 inch (maximum) guidewire. It is often necessary to introduce the device more than once and further down the epicardial artery on each successive pass to obtain optimal thrombus clearance and satisfactory TIMI grade 3 flow.

In circumstances with significant thrombus burden, adjunctive glycoprotein IIb/IIIa platelet receptor antagonist therapy will also aid in preventing subacute vessel closure and in reducing post-procedural complications,[2] by inhibiting thrombus regeneration and limiting distal embolization, especially if residual thrombus deposits are still visible angiographically.

References

1. Tofler GH. Triggering and the pathophysiology of acute coronary syndromes. *Am J Heart* 1997; **134**:S55–S61.

2. The EPIC Investigators. Use of a monoclonal antibody directed against the platelet glycoprotein IIb/IIIa receptor in high-risk coronary angioplasty. *N Engl J Med* 1994; **330**:956–61.

Case 16

TREATMENT OF ACUTE MYOCARDIAL INFARCTION (AMI) WITH EMBOLUS ASPIRATION

Vassilis Spanos, Carlo Di Mario and Michele Opizzi

Background

A 58-year-old patient with systemic hypertension, paroxysmal atrial fibrillation (AF), previous stent implantation in the mid-left anterior descending (LAD) 2 years before, treated with diltiazem and aspirin.

Chief complaint

Two days before the patient experienced a prolonged episode (32 hours) of tachyarrhythmia, which was well tolerated with spontaneous cessation. About 45 minutes before hospital admission the patient experienced severe chest pain which radiated to both arms with ST–T changes in the anterior and inferior leads (Fig. 16.1a). This resulted in immediate referral to the catheter laboratory.

Coronary angiography

LAD: Patent stent with minimal hyperplasia in the mid-segment; total blunt occlusion of the distal LAD without evident contrast staining (Figs. 16.2a and b). No significant lesions in the left circumflex (LCx) and the right coronary artery (RCA) without collaterals to the distal LAD.

Percutaneous treatment

Selective intracoronary thrombolysis

Six French (Fr) XB Zuma Medtronic guiding catheter; 0.014 inch Guidant BMW guidewire easily inserted to the distal LAD (apex); prolonged infusion

(30 minutes) of 900 000 IU urokinase via a Tracker 3.5 Fr infusion catheter positioned initially proximal to and then passed through the occlusion. No electrocardiographic (EC) or angiographic changes.

Balloon angioplasty

A Ranger balloon (2.0 mm; Boston Scientific) was advanced distally to the lesion and distal flow was followed with selective injection via the over-the-wire balloon catheter. The wire was reinserted and multiple balloon dilatations were performed through the occluded segment at 6 atmospheres. There was no indentation of the balloon and no angiographic changes; there was a transient increase in chest pain and ST elevation.

Thrombus aspiration

The guiding catheter was changed to an 8 Fr Cordis XB 3.5; the wire was readvanced and two passes of a 4.5 Fr Boston Scientific RESCUE catheter connected to a vacuum pump were performed (Fig. 16.3). A small amount of ruby-red thrombus was collected in the filter of the suction circuit. There was complete resolution of the occlusion with no residual narrowing and normal TIMI grade 3 flow (Figs 16.2c and d).

Clinical outcome

There was a rapid resolution of chest pain and ST elevation (Fig. 16.1b), with a maximum creatine kinase (CK) increase of 545 IU/l. The trans-esophageal ECG showed no left atrial thrombi and hypokinesia of the left ventricular (LV) apex. The patient was discharged after 3 days of uneventful hospital stay. Anticoagulation with warfarin was started before discharge and radiofrequency ablation of the left atrium, guided by left atrial mapping with the CARTO system,[1] was planned. There had been no recurrent episodes of paroxysmal AF after 3 months.

Discussion

Coronary embolism is a rare but well-recognized cause of AMI. It commonly involves the distal branches of the LAD coronary artery.[2] It is more frequent in patients with prosthetic valves or endocarditis, but it can be also caused

86

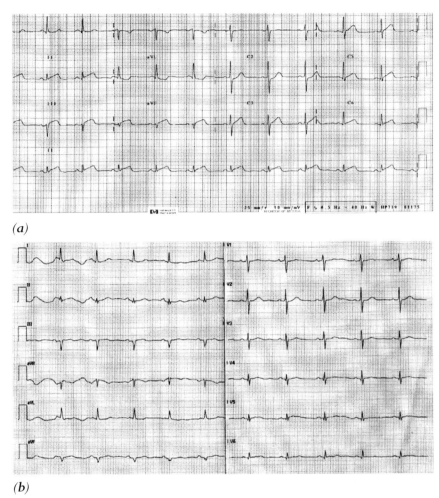

(a)

(b)

Figure 16.1. *(a) ECG after patient admission shows the presence of ST-segment elevation in V_4–V_6 and in D_2–D_3 and aVF. (b) Two hours after the end of PTCA, there is almost complete resolution of the ECG changes.*

by left atrial myxoma or thrombi. There are also cases due to paradoxical emboli or iatrogenic causes.[2,3]

AF, including paroxysmal AF, has been reported in patients with coronary emboli and a baseline condition of mitral stenosis,[4] and is a well-known cause of systemic emboli due to thrombi, typically in the left atrial appendage, with a risk of embolic stroke (3.2%/year) in patients taking aspirin.[5,6]

The AMI caused by coronary emboli presents *a therapeutic challenge*, since the thrombus is already organized and, for this reason, is usually resistant to

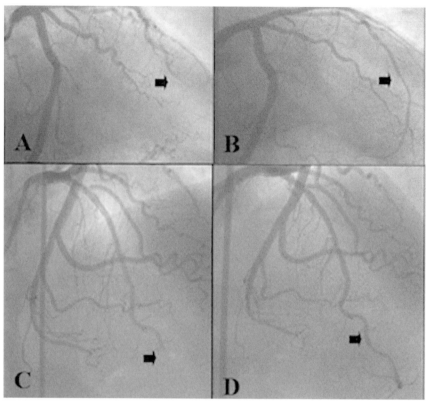

Figure 16.2. *Selective left coronary angiogram in the right oblique view* (**a**) *and cranial view* (**c**) *before treatment. Note the complete occlusion of the distal LAD with no filling of the distal third of the vessel. After thrombus aspiration* (**b**) *and* (**d**) *in the same views show complete restoration of flow and no stenosis or residual filling defect at the site of occlusion.*

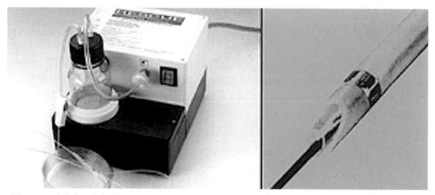

Figure 16.3. (**a**) *Low pressure vacuum pump of the Boston Scientific RESCUE system.* (**b**) *Dual lumen 4.5 Fr aspiration catheter.*

thrombolytic treatment (systemic or intracoronary). The conventional interventional approach can prove ineffective or harmful, since any gain after plain old balloon angioplasty (POBA) is jeopardized by early recoil, and the thrombi can prolapse and eventually embolize through the stent struts. It is also unlikely that these platelet-free old thrombi respond favorably to new agents, such as the glycoprotein IIb/IIIa receptor inhibitors.

This case elucidated all these problems in the first phase of the treatment and demonstrated that thrombectomy or thrombus aspiration is required to restore normal flow.

The RESCUE catheter (Boston Scientific) is a 4.5 Fr dual lumen monorail catheter, able to aspirate thrombi after connection to a low-pressure pump (Fig. 16.3). The large size of the device is an obvious limitation, but it allows aspiration of large thrombi without fragmentation and distal embolization. A wide range of alternative devices are used in the interventional treatment of thrombi: catheter-based high-power, low-frequency ultrasound leads to thrombus cavitation and fragmentation (Acolysis; Angiosonics Inc.); the Transluminal Extraction Catheter (TEC; Interventional Technologies); the new (CE marked in June 1999) X-Sizer device (EndiCOR Medical Inc.); the Possis Angiojet (Possis Medical) and the Cordis Hydrolyzer (Cordis Corp.) are hydrodynamic thrombectomy catheters which operate on the Venturi principle. These systems have been successfully used in the treatment of thrombus-containing lesions,[7–9] but their therapeutic potential is constrained in the setting of already organized thrombi (formed 24–48 hours before device insertion), as is usually the case with AMI caused by an embolus.

References

1. Pappone C, Oreto G, Vicedomini G et al. Catheter ablation of paroxysmal atrial fibrillation using a 3D mapping system. *Circulation* 1999; **100**:1203–8.

2. Braunwald E. *Heart Disease. A Textbook of Cardiovascular Medicine*, 5th edn. (WB Saunders: Philadelphia, 1997).

3. Cheng TO. Coronary embolism. *Am Heart J* 1996; **132**:1314–16.

4. Reddy CR, Ramakrishma Reddy M et al. Coronary embolism in mitral stenosis. *Indian Heart J* 1969; **21**:233–40.

5. Stroke Prevention in Atrial Fibrillation Investigators. Prospective identification of patients with nonvalvular atrial fibrillation at low-risk of stroke during treatment with aspirin. *J Am Med Assoc* 1998; **279**:1273–7.

89

6. Robert G, Hart M, Lesly A et al. Stroke with intermittent atrial fibrillation: incidence and predictors during aspirin therapy. *J Am Coll Cardiol* 2000; **35**:183–7.

7. Belli G, Pezzano A, Klugmann S et al. Adjunctive thrombus aspiration and mechanical protection from distal embolization in primary percutaneous intervention for acute myocardial infarction. *Cathet Cardiovasc Intervent* 2000 **50**:362–70.

8. Rosenschein U, Roth A, Rassin T et al. Analysis of coronary ultrasound thrombolysis endpoints in acute myocardial infarction (ACUTE trial). Results of the feasibility phase. *Circulation* 1997; **95**:1411–16.

9. Rodes J, Bilodeau L. Angioscopic evaluation of thrombus removal by the POSSIS AngioJet thrombectomy catheter. *Cathet Cardiovasc Diagn* 1998; **43**:338–43.

Case 17

A PATIENT WITH ACUTE MYOCARDIAL INFARCTION (AMI) AND INTRACORONARY CONTRAST FILLING DEFECT

Michael Haude, Holger Eggebrecht, Clemens von Birgelen, Thomas Budde and Raimund Erbel

Background

A 57-year-old male patient underwent coronary angiography in October 1999 because of angina pectoris class CCS III. Two-vessel disease (2VD) was documented with involvement of the left circumflex artery (LCx) and of the proximal left anterior descending (LAD) artery at the site of the origin of the first diagonal branch (D1), which itself presented an ostial stenosis. In this session the patient received a 3.0 × 18 mm stent implantation in the LCx stenosis and bifurcation stenting of the LAD/diagonal branch stenoses. A 3.0 × 18 mm stent was implanted in the LAD stenosis and a 2.5 × 13 mm stent in the ostial stenosis of the diagonal branch. All stent implantations were performed at 14 atmospheres pressure. A kissing-balloon dilatation of the stents in the LAD and the diagonal branch was not performed. In addition, no intravascular ultrasound (IVUS) imaging was applied. Afterwards the patient received antithrombotic therapy with acetyl salicyclic acid 100 mg/day indefinitely and clopidogrel 300 mg loading dose and 75 mg/day for 4 weeks. Three days after this procedure the patient again complained about angina without significant electrocardiogram (ECG) changes. Because of suspected stent thrombosis, recatheterization was performed, which documented vessel patency.

This patient was free from angina until 3 months later in January 2000, when he developed unstable angina pectoris. On January 29, he developed severe angina pectoris for 3 hours. The patient presented himself at the hospital where he had received his stent implantation. On arrival, he developed ventricular fibrillation with consecutive defibrillation and required cardiopulmonary resuscitation. After stabilization, the recorded ECG showed ST-segment elevations in leads V1–V4 (Fig. 17.1). Despite mechanical resuscitation, thrombolytic therapy was initiated in the presence of

ST-segment elevation myocardial infarction, because there was no availability of an emergency catheterization service. The patient received rtPA and abciximab IV. During the next 2 hours, ST-segment elevations did not change but the patient's hemodynamic status deteriorated and he went into cardiogenic shock. Therefore, the patient was transferred to a hospital with facilities for emergency coronary interventions.

Cardiac catheterization

After hemodynamic stabilization, coronary angiography documented vessel patency of the right (RCA) and left (LCA) coronary arteries. In the right anterior oblique (RAO) projection there was a persisting contrast filling defect within the LAD stent just proximal to the origin of diagonal branch (Fig. 17.2a), which was not present in the left anterior oblique (LAO) projection (Fig. 17.2b). The distal LAD appeared very tiny. The RCA showed no significant stenoses (Fig. 17.2c). Contrast medium flow was TIMI grade 3 flow in all coronary artery segments. Left ventricular (LV) angiography revealed anterior dyskinesia (Fig. 17.3).

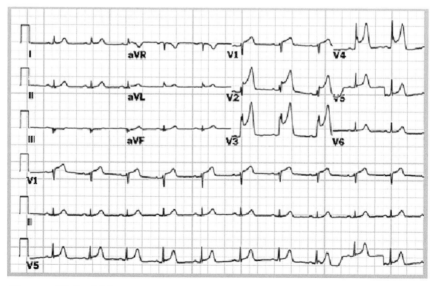

Figure 17.1. ECG.

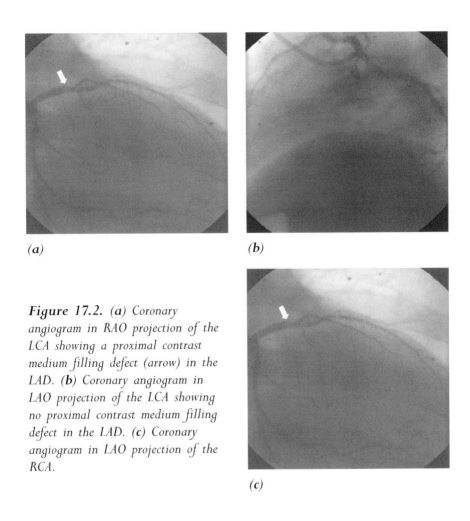

(a)

(b)

Figure 17.2. (a) Coronary angiogram in RAO projection of the LCA showing a proximal contrast medium filling defect (arrow) in the LAD. (b) Coronary angiogram in LAO projection of the LCA showing no proximal contrast medium filling defect in the LAD. (c) Coronary angiogram in LAO projection of the RCA.

(c)

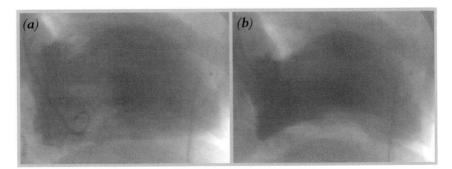

Figure 17.3. LV angiography in (a) diastole and (b) end systole.

93

Questions

- What is the cause of the contrast medium filling defect?
  Potential explanations are a local thrombus formation, a significant calcium deposit in the vessel wall, a contrast medium flow artifact or side-branch superposition.
- What are the potential options?

IVUS imaging

In order to evaluate the cause of the contrast filling defect in the LAD stent we performed an intracoronary ultrasound pullback study (Endosonics, Vision 5), from distal to proximal (Fig. 17.4). The cross-sectional images documented a complete stent strut apposition distal to the origin of the diagonal branch with a minimal lumen area (MLA) of $4.91\,\mathrm{mm}^2$. Proximal to the origin of the diagonal branch, the lumen size of the LAD increased significantly, to an MLA of $14.52\,\mathrm{mm}^2$, and the proximal end of the stent was completely hanging in the lumen without any apposition of the struts (Fig. 17.5). There were no intraluminal masses, suggesting the presence of thrombus burden, nor significant vessel wall calcifications. Therefore, we

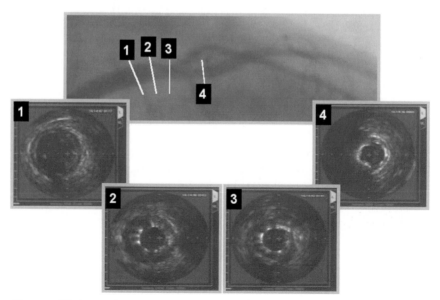

Figure 17.4. *IVUS cross-sectional images of the proximal LAD.*

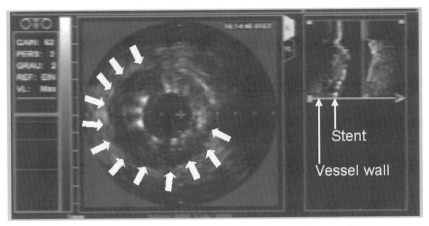

Figure 17.5. *IVUS cross-sectional image of the proximal LAD showing a completely underexpanded proximal end of the stent with no apposition to the vessel wall (arrows).*

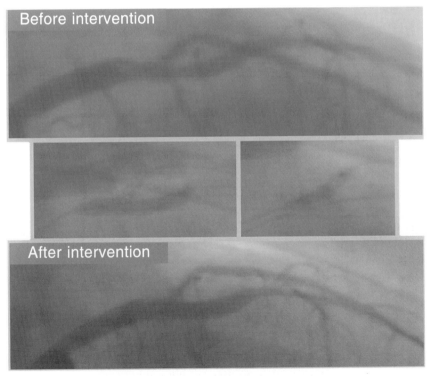

Figure 17.6. *Coronary angiograms before and after percutaneous transluminal coronary angioplasty (PTCA) of the underexpanded stent in the LAD and in the ostial stent of the diagonal branch.*

95

interpreted the persisting angiographic contrast filling defect in the proximal LAD stent segment as a contrast flow artifact caused by the underdeployed stent mesh tube. In addition, we concluded that this underdeployed stent caused stent thrombosis, and was the reason for the AMI with consecutive ventricular fibrillation and resuscitation. At the time of the catheterization this thrombus had dissolved because of the administration of thrombolytics and glycoprotein IIb/IIIa blocker agents.

Therapeutic strategy

Based on the findings of the IVUS study and the consecutive interpretations it was decided to dilate the LAD stent to achieve complete proximal stent strut apposition (Fig. 17.6). In addition, the stent in the origin of the diagonal branch was dilated. The final angiographic result showed no contrast medium filling defect, with persisting TIMI grade 3 flow to the distal LAD and the diagonal branch. The repeat IVUS study (Fig. 17.7) documented a complete proximal stent strut apposition to the vessel wall with a tapered distal stent conduit in the LAD.

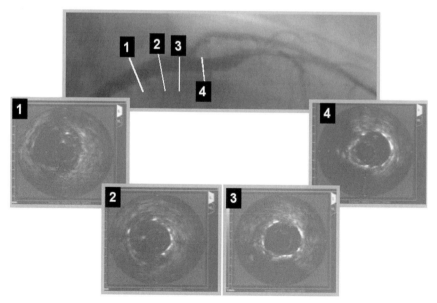

Figure 17.7. IVUS cross-sectional images of the proximal LAD after balloon angioplasty showing good stent strut apposition to the vessel wall.

Patient follow-up

During the next few days the patient presented several bleeding complications due to the combined thrombolytic and glycoprotein IIb/IIIa blocker therapy and mechanical resuscitation, including pulmonary and cerebral hemorrhage. The patient survived and could leave the hospital 6 weeks later without significant disability.

Conclusion

This case demonstrates the diagnostic value of IVUS for the evaluation of a contrast medium filling defect during anterior AMI because of suspected stent thrombosis.

Case 18

RECENT STENT OCCLUSION: SUCCESSFUL USE OF X-SIZER THROMBECTOMY

Thomas A Ischinger

Background

A 50-year-old male patient was admitted for unstable angina which had started 2 days earlier. The patient had received a stent in the proximal left anterior descending (LAD) 2 months previously. The electrocardiogram (ECG) showed signs of non-Q-wave myocardial infarction in the anterior leads. High-grade LAD restenosis, or functional occlusion, was suspected and acute coronary angiography was performed using the 5 French (Fr) Judkins technique.

Diagnostic angiogram

Coronary angiography revealed total occlusion of the LAD just proximal to the stent (Fig. 18.1a). The left circumflex (LCx) artery and the right coronary artery (RCA) had no relevant disease. Collaterals from the RCA filled the LAD retrogradely up to the proximal segment adjacent to the distal end of the occluded LAD stent.

The patient had been on aspirin 100 mg and was given a weight-adjusted dose of unfractionated heparin at completion of the diagnostic angiogram.

Treatment and rationale

Given the recent onset of symptoms, the occlusion was assumed to be relatively fresh and thrombotic, probably overlying a restenotic process. Therefore, it was decided to use a thrombectomy device, in this case an X-Sizer catheter (4.5 Fr), for three reasons: (a) minimization of the risk of

99

distal embolization associated with balloon dilatation in thrombotic lesions; (b) expeditious restoration of flow and; (c) creation of a sufficiently large thrombus-free lumen for adjunct and final measures (balloon/stent).

The X-Sizer thrombectomy catheter is a catheter using suction and rotation of an Archimedes screw at the distal tip to remove soft tissue from coronary vessels (Fig. 18.1b). It comes with a hand-held battery-powered motor unit and a vacuum container for suction and collection of removed debris. Priming takes minutes and the system is introduced over conventional 0.014 inch guidewires and through conventional percutaneous transluminal coronary angioplasty (PTCA) guide catheters (8 or 7 Fr, but recently 6 Fr, compatible).

Procedure

Using an 8 Fr guide catheter (Cordis, FL4) the occlusion was easily passed with an 0.014 inch standard wire, confirming the soft character of the occlusion. After extension of the wire, the activated X-Sizer was advanced through the occlusion with minimal resistance (Fig. 18.1b). Three passes were performed. The angiogram after removal of the X-sizer showed TIMI grade 3 flow (Fig. 18.1c). Residual stenosis was present; however, no relevant improvement was achieved with final balloon dilatation (Fig. 18.1d). There was no embolization and no enzyme rise. Two debris particles retrieved from the vacuum container after the procedure were histologically identified as 2–3 day old thrombus (Fig. 18.2).

An abciximab bolus was given after X-Sizer use and infusion was continued until the next day. Aspirin 100 mg and clopidogrel 75 mg (for 4 weeks) were continued. The patient remained asymptomatic over 6 months follow-up.

Commentary

Thrombus remains a major challenge in interventional cardiology, despite advanced technologies and powerful antithrombotic strategies, including lysis and glycoprotein IIb/IIIa antagonists. Lesions with thrombus are often resistant to balloon dilatation and have a propensity to reocclude, fragment or embolize, and are therefore associated with reduced success and increased complication rates in native coronaries and, in particular, in occluded vein

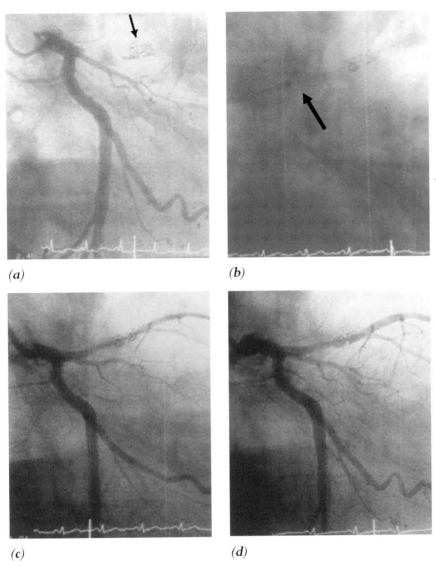

Figure 18.1. (a) Occluded LAD proximal to stent (arrow). (b) Advancement of X-Sizer over 0.014 inch wire to stent. (c) Antegrade flow (TIMI grade 3) after two passes. (d) No further improvement with final balloon dilatation.

grafts.[1–3] Pharmacological measures may take longer than mechanical procedures to be effective. Debulking lesions with thrombus burden using thrombectomy devices may represent an effective treatment in selected patients for prompt restoration of TIMI grade 2–3 flow, and preparation of

101

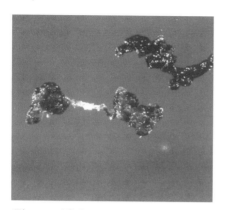

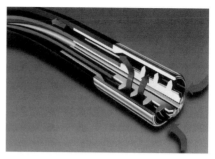

Figure 18.3. *Schematic of distal tip of X-Sizer containing rotating Archimedes screw.*

Figure 18.2. *Lemon-seed-sized particles retrieved from the vacuum container (2-day old thrombus).*

the vascular bed for balloon and stents. The X-Sizer is a safe, efficacious and relatively atraumatic device, with the rotation tip being blunt and contained within the distal end of the highly flexible catheter (Fig. 18.3). Small French-size, simplicity of set-up and ease of use make the X-Sizer a potentially helpful treatment option in settings with suspected or evident thrombus.[4]

References

1. Ellis SG, Roubin GS, King SB et al. Angiographic and clinical predictors of acute closure after native vessel coronary angioplasty. *Circulation* 1988; **77**:372–9.

2. Holmes DR, Berger PB. Percutaneous revascularization of occluded vein grafts: is it still a temptation to be resisted? (editorial). *Circulation* 1999; **99**:8–11.

3. Ahmad T, Webb JG, Carere RR, Dodek A. Coronary stenting for acute myocardial infarction. *Am J Cardiol* 1995; **76**:77–80.

4. Ischinger TA. Thrombectomy with the X-Sizer catheter system in the coronary circulation: initial results from a multicenter study. *J Invas Cardiol* 2002, in press.

Case 19

SUCCESSFUL THROMBECTOMY IN SEVERELY DISEASED VEIN GRAFT PRIOR TO STENT PLACEMENT

Thomas A Ischinger

Background

A 58-year-old male patient was admitted with onset of angina at rest 2 days earlier and prolonged pain on the day of admission. The patient had had a quadruple coronary artery bypass graft (CABG) 8 years previously [vein grafts to the right coronary artery (RCA) and diagonal branch, right internal mammary artery (RIMA) to the left circumflex (LCx) and left internal mammary artery (LIMA) to left anterior descending (LAD)]. Due to left bundle branch block, the electrocardiogram (ECG) could not be interpreted for ischemia; enzymes upon admission had remained negative. A coronary angiogram 1 year previously had shown moderate stenosis in the body of the RCA graft, an occluded RIMA to the LCx and a moderate stenosis in the vein graft to the diagonal branch, which was successfully treated by percutaneous transluminal coronary angioplasty. The patient had known obstructive lung disease, severe peripheral artery disease and a previous aortofemoral bypass.

Diagnostic angiography

Acutely performed repeat angiography revealed a patent LIMA to the LAD (small supply area), 75% irregular stenosis in the RCA graft and a functionally occluded graft to the diagonal branch with complex atherothrombotic disease in the ostial and mid-/distal segments. The native arteries were functionally occluded and not suitable for any catheter-based procedure. The left ventricular (LV) angiogram showed significant reduction of global LV ejection fraction (EF) to 35%, with extensive hypokinesis in the anterolateral and inferior walls. The condition of the patient worsened during angiography and diuretics; catecholamines and oxygen were needed.

103

Treatment and rationale

It was decided that expeditious reperfusion of the anterolateral wall (diagonal branch) would most likely help interrupt the development of cardiogenic shock. However, the thrombotic and degenerated appearance of the graft to the diagonal branch posed a major risk of distal embolization at the conventional balloon dilatation and stent implantation site. Therefore, thrombectomy using the X-Sizer catheter system as a prelude to stent implantation was chosen.

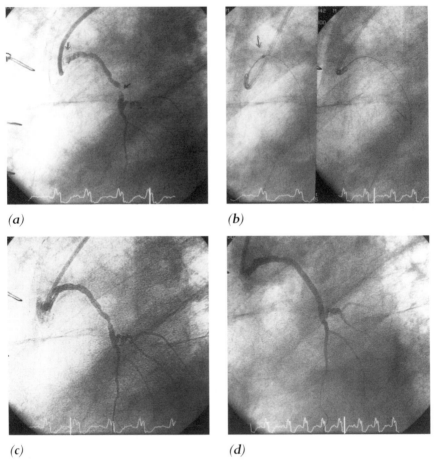

(a)   *(b)*

(c)   *(d)*

Figure 19.1. (a) *Angiogram of vein graft to diagonal branch with severe complex thrombotic lesions at ostium and in the distal segment (arrows).* (b) *X-Sizer catheter being advanced through vein graft (arrows indicate tip).* (c) *After two X-Sizer catheter passes. Graft partially cleared.* (d) *After placement of a 3.0 × 16 mm stent distally and a 3.5 × 15 mm stent at ostium.*

104

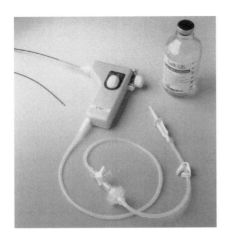

Figure 19.2. *X-Sizer catheter system with vacuum container and motor unit.*

Procedure

A 7 French (Fr) El Gamal guide catheter was positioned and an 0.014 inch extra support Galeo (Biotronik) guidewire passed through the graft stenoses into the distal diagonal branch. Two passes with the X-Sizer 1.5 mm catheter were performed along the entire length of the graft and multiple passes through the graft ostium. Angiography after the X-Sizer passes revealed a 'cleaned' graft appearance, permitting stent placements. A 3.0 × 16 mm Devon stent was placed in the distal segment and a 3.5 × 15 mm Prolink stent in the ostium of the graft. Final angiography showed excellent results in both segments. No distal embolization was noticed and no complications occurred. At the onset of the procedure, weight-adjusted heparin [unfractionated heparinization (UFH)] was given as was a bolus of eptifibatide with subsequent infusion for 24 hours and low-dose concomitant heparin. The sheath was pulled under eptifibatide infusion. The total procedure time was 25 minutes.

Enzymes (including troponin) remained negative. The patient was ambulatory on day 2 after the procedure, awaiting stent placement into the RCA graft.

Commentary

The single-use X-Sizer catheter system combines suction, by vacuum container, and rotation, of an Archimedes screw, for removal of atherothrombotic material from coronary arteries and vein grafts. The small catheter version (1.5 mm tip diameter) is 6 Fr guide-catheter compatible (an

105

8 Fr guide for a 2.0 mm tip). The system is driven by a hand-held battery-powered motor unit. It is primed within minutes and is introduced over conventional 0.014 inch guidewires using conventional angioplasty techniques.

Thrombus remains a major challenge in interventional cardiology, despite advanced technologies and novel antithrombotic strategies including glycoprotein IIb/IIIa antagonists. In this case, removal of loose and thrombotic material prior to balloon dilatation and stenting appeared warranted: lesions with thrombus, in particular in old vein grafts, carry a high risk of total occlusion and distal embolization during conventional catheter procedures. Expeditious debulking of lesions with thrombus burden by thrombectomy may represent a safe and effective treatment in certain patients, in particular those with ongoing ischemia, in order to achieve prompt restoration of TIMI grade 2–3 flow at reduced risk of embolization. Embolic protection devices may have been another treatment option; however, their use takes more time and the passage of the device through the risky target areas itself poses an embolization risk. Other (e.g. hydrodynamic) thrombectomy devices may serve the same purpose, yet need more preparation, hardware and larger guide catheters. The small French size, the flexibility, the simplicity of use and the safety profile (blunt rotating tip contained within the distal catheter tip) made the X-Sizer catheter the first choice in this case. The excellent result confirmed our decision.

Further reading

Holmes DR, Berger PB. Percutaneous revascularization of occluded vein grafts: is it still a temptation to be resisted? *Circulation* 1999; **99**:8–11.

Ischinger TA. Thrombectomy with the X-Sizer catheter system in the coronary circulation: initial results from a multicenter study. *J Invas Cardiol* 2002; **13**:81–8.

Mak KH, Callapalli R, Eisenberg MJ et al. Effect of platelet glycoprotein IIb/IIIa receptor inhibition on distal embolization during percutaneous revascularization of aortocoronary saphenous vein grafts. EPIC investigators. *Am J Cardiol* 1997; **80**:985–8.

Case 20

Combined Stenting Of A Degenerated Saphenous Vein Graft (SVG) And A Native Coronary Artery In One Session With A Protective Device

Talib K Majwal

Background

Diffusely degenerated SVG (defined as >3 years old SVG and lesion >20 mm in length) carry a challenge to the interventional cardiologist, particularly as thrombus has been observed in 70% of old grafts by angioscopy.

The two major limitations of percutaneous coronary intervention (PCI) in degenerated SVG are the risk of distal embolization and poor long-term outcomes.

Case report

A 65-year-old male with no history of hypertension or diabetes mellitus and with normal serum lipids underwent coronary artery bypass surgery (CABG) 15 years previously, with SVG to the left anterior descending (LAD) artery, the first marginal artery (OM1) (Fig. 20.1) and to the distal right coronary artery (RCA).

The patient was stable until recently, when he presented with unstable angina class IIB2. The electrocardiogram (ECG) showed old inferior myocardial infarction.

Angiography revealed 80% stenosis in the mid-LAD, total OM1 occlusion, 90% stenosis in the circumflex (Cx) to OM2, total RCA occlusion and the left ventricular (LV) ejection fraction (EF) was 49%.

107

SVG to the RCA showed severe stenosis in the mid-part of the graft body with a filling defect distal to the stenosis (Fig. 20.2); the SVG to OM1 showed 80% stenosis with small filling defects (Fig. 20.3) and patent SVG to the LAD.

The patient received clopidogrel 75 mg and ASA 325 mg daily 3 days prior to intervention.

Using a 7 French (Fr) multipurpose guiding catheter, PCI of the SVG to the RCA was undertaken by passing a 6 mm Angioguard (Cordis Corp., Miami Lakes, FL) distal to the lesion (Fig. 20.4); direct stenting (DS) was then undertaken with a 4.0 × 23 mm Bx Velocity stent (Cordis) up to 10 atmospheres with a good result (Fig. 20.5). No complications were observed but a small quantity of debris was removed from the Angioguard.

The same guiding catheter was used to cannulate the SVG to OM1, and a second 6 mm Angioguard advanced beyond the stenosis (Fig. 20.6) followed by DS with a 4.0 × 18 mm Bx Velocity stent up to 9 atmospheres with a good result (Fig. 20.7). No complications were observed.

The procedure ended with stenting of the native Cx to OM2, with a 2.7 × 13 mm Bx Velocity (Cordis) stent after balloon predilation (Fig. 20.8).

Six months clinical follow-up was uneventful, the patient being symptom free.

There are several types of catheter-based systems designed to prevent distal embolization which may prevent the no-reflow phenomenon. The results of ongoing multicenter studies show good and promising results.

In this case it was thought that the use of a protective device in 15-year-old degenerated grafts was essential, especially in the presence of filling defects. The use of this device may explain why this patient experienced no distal embolization and no reflow, and was without myocardial enzyme elevation.

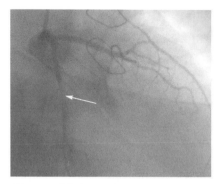

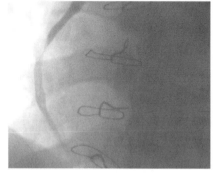

Figure 20.1. Right anterior oblique (RAO) projection: shows stenosis of left Cx to OM2 (white arrow).

Figure 20.2. Left anterior oblique (LAO) projection: SVG to the distal RCA shows severe stenosis with a filling defect and diminished flow distally.

108

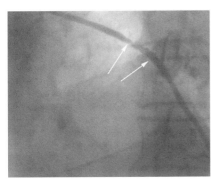

Figure 20.3. *LAO projection: SVG to OM1, 80% stenosis with a small filling defect.*

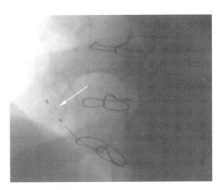

Figure 20.4. *Expanded Angioguard protective device in the SVG to the RCA (white arrow).*

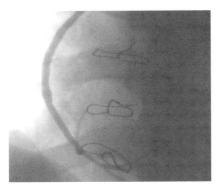

Figure 20.5. *LAO projection: SVG to the distal RCA; good final result after stenting and good distal run-off.*

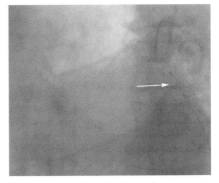

Figure 20.6. *Expanded Angioguard protective device in the SVG to OM1 (white arrow).*

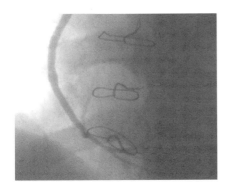

Figure 20.7. *LAO projection: SVG to OM1; good final result after stenting.*

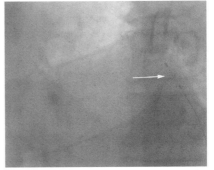

Figure 20.8. *RAO projection: native left Cx to OM2 after stenting with 2.75 × 13 mm stent.*

109

Case 21

STENT THROMBOSIS SOON AFTER NON-CARDIAC SURGERY

Andrew Farb, Joseph P Lindsay Jr and Renu Virmani

Background

A 71-year-old black man with coronary atherosclerosis and mildly reduced left ventricular (LV) function was admitted for removal of 7 mm of left lower lobe lung nodule. Preoperatively, an isotope cardiac stress demonstrated myocardial ischemia, but the patient was not having cardiac symptoms. Coronary angiography was performed which revealed a 90% diameter stenosis in the proximal left anterior descending (LAD) coronary artery. The distal LAD was occluded with good collateral flow from a non-dominant right coronary artery (RCA). A 95% lumen diameter stenosis was present in the proximal ramus intermedius (RI) artery. The proximal LAD lesion was predilated followed by placement of two overlapping 3.0 × 15 mm Multi-Link Duet stents deployed at 14 atmospheres balloon pressure for 14 and 22 seconds. The stenosis was reduced to 0%. An attempt to cross the ramus lesion with a guidewire was unsuccessful. There were no complications related to the coronary intervention, and the patient was placed on aspirin and clopidogrel.

Antiplatelet therapy was stopped, and thoracotomy and lung wedge resection were performed 5 days post-coronary stent placement. Pathologic analysis of the resected portion of the left lower lobe demonstrated focal pulmonary scarring without a neoplasm being present. On postoperative day 1, the patient developed confusion and respiratory distress, followed by cardiac arrest. An autopsy was performed.

Angiographic and radiographic commentary

There was a 90% diameter stenosis of the proximal LAD coronary beginning at its ostium (Fig. 21.1a). Post-stent deployment (Fig. 21.1b), the stenosis was reduced to 0%. Post-mortem radiography (Fig. 21.1c) showed two

Multi-Link Duet stents in the heavily calcified proximal LAD coronary artery, just distal to the ostium of the RI, with a short overlapped segment of the stents (Fig. 21.1c).

Pathologic commentary

Examination of the coronary arteries showed severe atherosclerosis with focal marked calcification involving all three major epicardial arteries. There was an acute occlusive thrombus in the proximal portion of the first stent (near the origin of the RI) associated with fibrous cap disruption (with superficial extrusion of the lipid core into the lumen), focal plaque disruption and focal

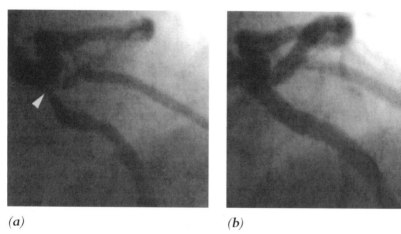

(a)   *(b)*

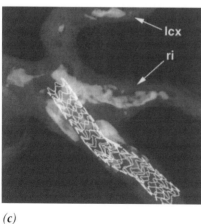

(c)

Figure 21.1. (a) A left anterior oblique (LAO) caudal view demonstrating a 90% diameter stenosis of the proximal LAD coronary artery (arrowhead) beginning at its ostium. (b) Post-stent deployment, the stenosis was reduced to 0%. (c) A post-mortem radiograph shows two overlapping Multi-Link Duet stents in the heavily calcified proximal LAD coronary artery, just distal to the ostium of the calcified RI (ri). The left circumflex artery is indicated (lcx).

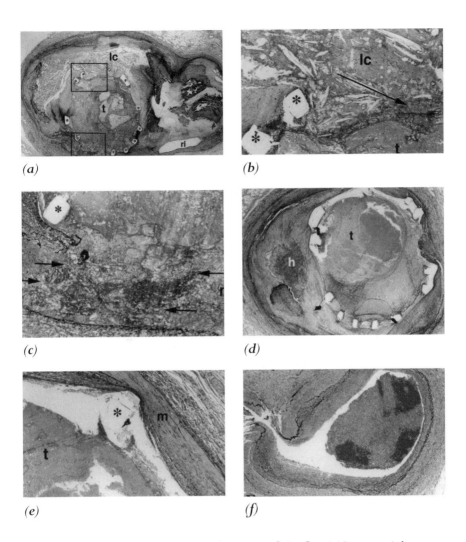

Figure 21.2. (a) The most proximal portion of the first LAD stent. A large lipid core (lc) is present. The ostium of the markedly calcified and stenotic (>95% narrowing) RI is seen to the right with the lumen of the RI indicated by 'ri'. The LAD stent struts are indicated by (*) and the stent lumen is occluded by an acute thrombus (t). (b) The upper box in (a) is magnified and shows rupture of the thin fibrous cap overlying the lipid core (arrow) with penetration of a stent strut into the core. The lower box in (c) is magnified in (a); focal medial (m) rupture is present between the arrows. (d) A section towards the middle of the first stent; a focally calcified and hemorrhagic (h) plaque is present, and the lumen is occluded by a thrombus (t). (e) A high-power view of a stent strut (*) compressing the arterial media (m). (f) A large thromboembolism in the LAD just distal to the stented arterial segment is shown.

medial rupture (Fig. 21.2a–e). Embolized thrombus was present in the arterial segment just distal to the second stent (Fig. 21.2f).

The myocardium demonstrated a transmural acute myocardial infarction (AMI) involving the interventricular septum and anterior wall (Fig. 21.3a). Histologic examination showed early myocyte coagulation necrosis and interstitial infiltration of neutrophils (Fig. 21.3b). Additionally, there was a healed, patchy subendocardial anterior and septal myocardial infarction.

Discussion

Preoperative assessment of coronary disease severity is a well-accepted practice for patients with risk factors for atherosclerosis undergoing non-cardiac surgery. Patients at particularly high cardiovascular risk associated with non-cardiac surgery are those with unstable coronary artery syndromes, decompensated heart failure, significant arrhythmias and severe valvular heart disease.[1] Patients at intermediate risk are those with mild angina, prior myocardial infarction, compensated heart failure and diabetes mellitus.[1] Retrospective studies have suggested that patients treated with prior coronary artery bypass (CABG) surgery have improved survival compared to medically-managed patients;[2,3] e.g. in the Coronary Artery Surgery Study (CASS) registry, postoperative mortality was reduced from 3.3 to 1.7% and myocardial infarction from 2.7 to 0.8% in CABG-treated patients undergoing high-risk non-cardiac surgery.[4] The present general recommendation is to

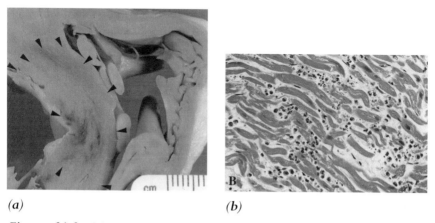

(a)   *(b)*

Figure 21.3. (a) *Gross heart, mid-ventricular slice, shows an acute transmural myocardial infarction of the anterior ventricular septum.* (b) *Histology demonstrates myocyte necrosis associated with interstitial neutrophil infiltrates.*

114

perform bypass surgery before non-cardiac surgery in those individuals who otherwise meet the established indications for CABG: left main coronary stenosis, three-vessel atherosclerosis with LV dysfunction, two-vessel coronary stenosis including severe LAD disease and intractable symptoms despite maximal medial therapy.[5]

The clinical benefit of preoperative percutaneous coronary revascularization is less assured compared with CABG performed before non-cardiac surgery. Several small retrospective studies have shown a low incidence of cardiac death in patients treated with preoperative balloon angioplasty (PTCA).[6–8] The clinical applicability of these data is circumscribed by their small sample size, retrospective analysis, and limited comparisons to medical treatment and CABG surgery. Further, other studies have not demonstrated a reduction in mortality in patients undergoing PTCA before non-cardiac surgery.[9,10]

Stent placement is currently employed in most catheter-based coronary interventions in the USA and is associated with improved clinical outcome versus PTCA. The risk of acute or subacute stent thrombosis in elective stent placement has largely been solved (<1% incidence) by improved stent deployment techniques that fully appose the stent to the vessel wall [via high-pressure balloon inflation with or without intravascular ultrasound (IVUS)] and more effective antiplatelet therapy (aspirin plus ticlopidine or clopidogrel).[11–14]

There are no prospective trials reporting on the use of prophylactic coronary stenting before non-cardiac surgery. However, recent data indicate a high risk of stent thrombosis after non-cardiac surgery performed soon after stenting.[15] In a study of 40 patients who underwent coronary artery stent placement <6 weeks before non-cardiac surgery requiring general anesthesia, there were seven myocardial infarctions, 11 major hemorrhages and eight deaths (20% of the study group). All infarcts and deaths occurred in patients undergoing surgery ≤11 days post-stent placement (mean 9 ± 3 days, range 1–11 days). Importantly, the withdrawal of antiplatelet therapy correlated with stent-related complications; of the nine patients with major complications (death, myocardial infarction or both), only one patient had not discontinued use of both aspirin and ticlopidine prior to surgery, two patients had only ticlopidine stopped, and six had both aspirin and ticlopidine withheld prior to surgery. The mechanism of AMI in these cases was probably stent thrombosis, which was confirmed angiographically in two patients and presumed based on electrocardiographic evidence of ischemia or infarction in four individuals.[15]

Notably, in the present case, the patient was asymptomatic despite the presence of severe coronary atherosclerosis and an abnormal exercise stress

115

test. From an interventional and morphologic standpoint, the stent deployment itself was technically well performed. The critical clinical decision was to stop antiplatelet therapy before a full course was administered and proceed with pulmonary surgery. Acute stent thrombosis occurred on the first postoperative day, leading to AMI and death. Local arterial morphologic factors also probably contributed to acute thrombosis in this case. The plaque was highly necrotic in its proximal portion with a large lipid core and thin fibrous cap. Balloon angioplasty and stent deployment resulted in fibrous cap rupture, leading to exposure of the thrombogenic lipid core to circulating blood. Other factors of less importance, but which may have contributed to stent thrombosis, include LAD stent location (which has the highest frequency of stent thrombosis among the coronary arteries) and compromised distal arterial run-off (secondary to occlusion of the distal LAD).

The mechanism of stent thrombosis after non-cardiac surgery is almost certainly related to premature discontinuation of antiplatelet therapy rather than suboptimal stent implant technique. In addition, catheter-based cardiac interventions and surgical procedures can stimulate the coagulation system and inflammatory responses, which can potentially lead to a prothrombotic state.[16]

The present case illustrates the potential hazards of premature discontinuation of aspirin and clopidogrel or ticlopidine followed by major surgery. In patients for whom preoperative catheter-based coronary revascularization is believed to be essential, PTCA alone, rather than stenting, should be considered because of the lower associated acute thrombotic risk. If surgery becomes urgent and coronary stenting is deemed necessary, clopidogrel and aspirin should be administered starting several days before stenting (if possible) and reinitiated as soon as possible postoperatively to complete at least a 14-day course. In all other cases, stenting is best avoided at least 30 days before non-cardiac surgery, especially if antiplatelet therapy needs to be interrupted.

References

1. ACC/AHA Task Force on Practice Guidelines. ACC/AHA guidelines for perioperative cardiovascular evaluation for noncardiac surgery. *Circulation* 1996; **93**:1280–317.

2. Foster ED, Davis KB, Carpenter JA et al. Risk of noncardiac operation in patients with defined coronary disease: the Coronary Artery Surgery Study (CASS) registry experience. *Ann Thorac Surg* 1986; **41**:42–50.

3. Hertzer NR, Young JR, Beven EG et al. Late results of coronary bypass in patients with peripheral vascular disease. II. Five-year survival according to sex, hypertension, and diabetes. *Cleve Clin J Med* 1987; **54**:15–23.

4. Eagle KA, Rihal CS, Mickel MC et al. Cardiac risk of noncardiac surgery: influence of coronary disease and type of surgery in 3368 operations. CASS Investigators and University of Michigan Heart Care Program. Coronary Artery Surgery Study. *Circulation* 1997; **96**:1882–7.

5. ACC/AHA guidelines and indications for coronary artery bypass graft surgery. A report of the American College of Cardiology/American Heart Association Task Force on Assessment of Diagnostic and Therapeutic Cardiovascular Procedures (Subcommittee on Coronary Artery Bypass Graft Surgery). *Circulation* 1991; **83**:1125–73.

6. Allen JR, Helling TS, Hartzler GO. Operative procedures not involving the heart after percutaneous transluminal coronary angioplasty. *Surg Gynecol Obstet* 1991; **173**:285–8.

7. Huber KC, Evans MA, Bresnahan JF et al. Outcome of noncardiac operations in patients with severe coronary artery disease successfully treated preoperatively with coronary angioplasty. *Mayo Clin Proc* 1992; **67**:15–21.

8. Elmore JR, Hallet Jr JW, Gibbons RJ et al. Myocardial revascularization before abdominal aortic aneurysmorrhaphy: effect of coronary angioplasty. *Mayo Clin Proc* 1993; **68**:637–41.

9. Mason JJ, Owens DK, Harris RA et al. The role of coronary angiography and coronary revascularization before noncardiac vascular surgery. *J Am Med Ass* 1995; **273**:1919–25.

10. Posner KL, Van Norman GA, Chan V. Adverse cardiac outcomes after noncardiac surgery in patients with prior percutaneous transluminal coronary angioplasty. *Anesth Analg* 1999; **89**:553–60.

11. Leon MB, Baim DS, Popma JJ et al. A clinical trial comparing three antithrombotic-drug regimens after coronary-artery stenting. Stent Anticoagulation Restenosis Study Investigators. *N Engl J Med* 1998; **339**:1665–71.

12. Jauhar R, Bergman G, Savino S et al. Effectiveness of aspirin and clopidogrel combination therapy in coronary stenting. *Am J Cardiol* 1999; **84**:726–8.

13. Berger PB, Bell MR, Rihal CS et al. Clopidogrel versus ticlopidine after intracoronary stent placement. *J Am Coll Cardiol* 1999; **34**:1891–4.

14. De Servi S, Repetto S, Klugmann S et al. Stent thrombosis: incidence and related factors in the RISE. Registry (Registro Impianto Stent Endocoronarico). *Cathet Cardiovasc Intervent* 1999; **46**:13–8.

15. Kaluza GL, Joseph J, Lee JR et al. Catastrophic outcomes of noncardiac surgery soon after coronary stenting. *J Am Coll Cardiol* 2000; **35**:1288–94.

16. Serrano Jr CV, Ramires JA, Venturinelli M et al. Coronary angioplasty results in leukocyte and platelet activation with adhesion molecule expression. Evidence of inflammatory responses in coronary angioplasty. *J Am Coll Cardiol* 1997; **29**:1276–83.

Case 22

GRAFT THROMBOSIS

Jochen Krämer, Rainer Dietz and C Michael Gross

Case report

Patient HH, a 40-year-old white female, presented in our emergency room with recent onset of typical unstable angina pectoris with radiation to the left arm. There was no dyspnea, pulmonary congestion or peripheral edema.

The electrocardiogram (ECG) at rest showed significant ischemia in the anterolateral and inferior leads with ST elevation and depression (Fig. 22.1) The cardiac enzymes 3 hours after the beginning of chest pain were positive [troponin T (TnT) 0.08 ng/ml; creatine kinase (CK) 150 U/l; CK myocardial band (MB) 29 U/l] and the coagulation parameters were as follows: PTT 56 seconds, TPZ 21%, with an INR of 3.7. The patient underwent emergency cardiac catheterization.

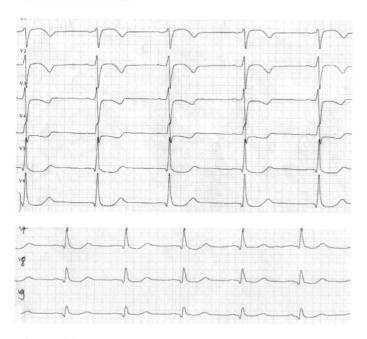

Figure 22.1.

119

The patient's medical history spanned more than 20 years, having previously been operated upon to correct (newly diagnosed) aortic isthmus stenosis in 1978. Throughout the 1980s, she had medical treatment for arterial hypertension, but was otherwise healthy.

In June 1999, she received an aortic valve prosthesis (Carbomedics 25 mm) with a Cabrol plastic graft (with reimplantation of the coronary arteries) due to aortic insufficiency (biscuspid valve, arterial hypertension, late-diagnosed aortic coarctation with consecutive aortic dilatation).

In October 2000, after a short period of angina pectoris and dyspnea on exertion, the patient underwent a coronary artery bypass graft (CABG) because all three vessels showed ostial lesions due to mechanical/ proliferative obstruction by the graft, and she received two arterial grafts [left internal mammary artery (LIMA) to the left anterior descending (LAD) artery and right internal mammary artery (RIMA) to the right coronary artery (RCA)], leaving the left circumflex (LCx) ungrafted. The usual care medication included metoprolol 100 mg and a coumarine derivate. The INR was documented to have been between 2.2 and 2.7 over the last few months.

Up to 1 week before admission, the patient felt healthy, then increasing shortness of breath on exertion developed.

After standard emergency medication (IV aspirin, heparin, nitroglycerin, morphine and metoprolol), the patient underwent coronary angiography. The coronary angiogram revealed a partly thrombosed Cabrol graft with a highly limited blood flow (TIMI grade 1 flow) into the LCx. Both arterial grafts were patent with a TIMI grade 3 flow. Due to an elevated INR, no glycoprotein IIb/IIIa antagonist was given.

Fig. 22.2 demonstrates the interventional procedure. The Cabrol graft and

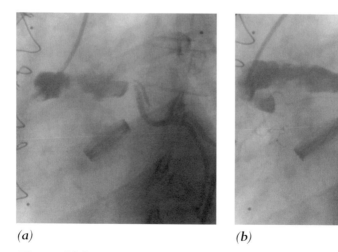

(a)   *(b)*

Figure 22.2.

120

the proximal LCx were filled with thrombus, leading to a reduced flow into the highly stenosed vessel (Fig. 22.2a); the LCx then was directly stented with a 3.5 mm stent, leading to a TIMI grade 3 flow (Fig. 22.2b).

Post-procedurally, the chest pain resolved and the patient recovered quickly. Cardiac enzymes raised only to a maximum of TnT 0.16 ng/ml, CK 285 U/l and CK-MB of 50 U/l 2 hours after admission; the ECG changes were completely resolved.

This case shows the necessity of a more aggressive anticoagulation therapy for patients having not only a mechanical valve but also a prosthesis like the Cabrol plastic graft. A coumarine derivate in a dose aiming for an INR of at least 3, aspirin 100 mg daily and clopidogrel 75 mg for 4 weeks were prescribed for this patient.

Case 23

MECHANICAL THROMBECTOMY

Christopher J White

Background

A 68-year-old man was admitted to hospital with a prolonged episode of chest pain and an elevated serum troponin level. His electrocardiogram (ECG) showed non-specific ST changes with evidence of an old inferior wall myocardial infarction. Due to recurrent episodes of pain, he was brought urgently to the cardiac catheterization laboratory for diagnostic angiography.

Angiography

Left ventriculography revealed a mildly abnormal left ventricular (LV) ejection fraction (EF) at 40% with inferior hypokinesis. The main left coronary artery (LCA) was patent. The left anterior descending (LAD) coronary artery was severely narrowed after the first septal perforator branch and the distal vessel filled from a patent left internal mammary bypass graft.

The right coronary artery (RCA) was occluded and the distal vessel filled via a patent saphenous vein graft (SVG) to the posterior descending artery. The native left circumflex (LCx) vessel was occluded at its origin and a distal obtuse marginal branch (OMB) filled via ipsilateral collaterals. Selective angiography of the SVG to the OMB demonstrated an occluded SVG with intraluminal filling defects (Fig. 23.1).

Mechanical thrombectomy using the Angiojet catheter (Possis, Minneapolis, MN) was the preferred technique to rapidly recanalize the culprit lesion. A temporary pacemaker was placed into the right ventricle via the right femoral vein. An 8 French (Fr) Hockey-stick (Medtronic, Minneapolis, MN) guiding catheter was advanced to engage the ostium of the vein graft and the total occlusion was crossed with a 260 cm long 0.014 inch extrasupport guidewire. The Angiojet catheter was advanced to the occlusion and activated as it was advanced slowly through the occlusion (Fig. 23.2). The Angiojet catheter was slowly withdrawn and readvanced across the lesion

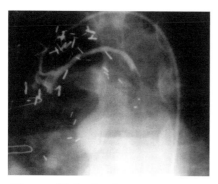

Figure 23.1. *Baseline angiogram [left anterior oblique (LAO) view] of the occluded SVG–OMB with angiographically visible thrombus.*

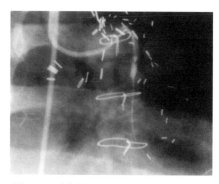

Figure 23.2. *Angiography [right anterior oblique (RAO) view] showing the Angiojet catheter in the lesion.*

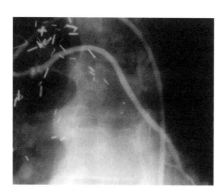

Figure 23.3. *Final angiogram (LAO view) after rheolytic thrombectomy and stent placement.*

several times. Angiography demonstrated marked luminal improvement with resolution of the filling defects; however, there was residual narrowing of the body of the graft. Three self-expanding Wallstents (Schneider, Watertown, MA) were placed end to end and then postdilated to ensure full apposition with the endoluminal surface of the graft (Fig. 23.3).

Commentary

The percutaneous approach to an occluded SVG lesion with a large clot burden is a complex and difficult issue. The first question to answer is whether this lesion should have been treated at all. The clinical impression was that this was definitely the culprit lesion causing the patient's recurrent ischemic symptoms.

124

The two most common treatment strategies for a thrombus containing lesion are intragraft thrombolysis,[1] or mechanical (rheolytic) thrombolysis[2] followed by definitive intervention. The recently completed VeGAS 2 trial compared an intragraft urokinase infusion to mechanical thrombectomy (Angiojet catheter) followed by definitive intervention, and demonstrated a safety and efficacy benefit in favor of mechanical thrombectomy.[2]

Rheolytic thrombectomy is an effective tool for the treatment of thrombus-containing SVG lesions. The system works by applying the Venturi–Bernoulli principle to aspirate intravascular thrombus. Three high-speed saline jets create a low-pressure region at the tip ($c.$ $-760\,mmHg$), which act to 'pull' the thrombus into the catheter exhaust lumen and propel it from the vessel.

One subset of the VeGAS 2 trial[2] included 188 patients with thrombus-containing lesions in SVG who were randomized either to mechanical thrombectomy with the Angiojet ($n = 97$) or an infusion of urokinase ($n = 91$). Major adverse coronary events (MACE) occurred in 23% of the Angiojet group versus 41% in the urokinase group ($P < 0.001$). Bleeding events and vascular complications were also significantly fewer in the Angiojet group.

In summary, the safety and efficacy of mechanical thrombectomy have been demonstrated in a randomized controlled trial to be superior to that of a local infusion of urokinase. This case is an example of the rapid and safe restoration of flow in thrombus-containing lesion treated with rheolytic thrombectomy followed by stent placement.

References

1. Hartmann JR, McKeever LS, O'Neill WW et al. Recanalization of chronically occluded aortocoronary saphenous vein bypass grafts with long term low dose direct infusion of urokinase: a serial trial (ROBUST). *J Am Coll Cardiol* 1996; **27**: 60–6.

2. Ramee SR, Baim DS, Popma JJ et al. A randomized prospective multicenter study comparing intracoronary urokinase to rheolytic thrombectomy with the Possis Angiojet Catheter for intracoronary thrombus: final result of the VeGAS 2 Trial. *Circulation* 1998; **98(Suppl I)**:I–86 (abstract).

Case 24

DETHROMBOSIS BY IV ADMINISTRATION OF ABCIXIMAB

Martin Oberhoff, Andreas Baumbach and Karl R Karsch

Background

A 37-year-old man with a history of coronary artery disease and a posterior infarct 1 year earlier was admitted to a general hospital with an acute anterior infarct. The electrocardiogram (ECG) on arrival demonstrated ST-segment elevation (2 mm) in the anterior leads (V2–V6). He received thrombolysis with rtPA [maximum creatine kinase (CK) 1824 IU/l]. Because he developed post-infarction angina he was admitted to our hospital for further investigation.

The angiogram showed apical, septal and anterior hypokinesia on ventriculography [ejection fraction (EF) 42%]. Coronary angiography (Figs 24.1a and b) revealed a three-vessel disease (3VD) with a moderate lesion in the right coronary artery (RCA) and a tight lesion in the mid-portion of the circumflex (Cx). The left anterior descending (LAD) artery showed a complex lesion with an intraluminal filling defect, including the origin of the first diagonal branch. The distal vessel was without significant disease. The patient was treated with an abciximab (ReoPro) bolus and 12-hour infusion, together with low-dose unfractionated heparin (UFH), and was investigated again the following day. This angiogram (Figs 24.2a and b) now showed an eccentric, circumscribed lesion, without the intraluminal filling defect previously seen proximal to the origin of the first diagonal branch (D1). The LAD lesion was treated by standard balloon angioplasty with a 3.5 mm balloon (9 atmospheres) with an excellent result.

Antagonists of the glycoprotein IIb/IIIa platelet receptors are very potent antithrombotic agents. Studies in patients scheduled for percutaneous coronary intervention (PCI) have shown that the administration of glycoprotein IIb/IIIa antagonists is associated with a reduction in death or myocardial infarction.[1,2] Experimental studies show that abciximab dramatically decreases mural thrombus formation after arterial injury.[3]

127

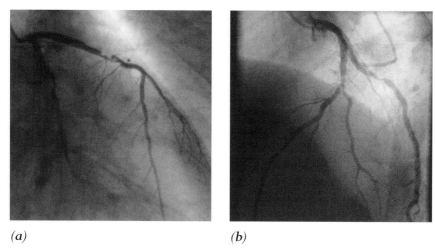

(a)   *(b)*

Figure 24.1. *Selective coronary angiograms of the left coronary artery (LCA) in (**a**) right anterior oblique (RAO) and (**b**) left anterior oblique (LAO) projections. There is a complex lesion in the LAD with an intraluminal filling defect including the origin of D1.*

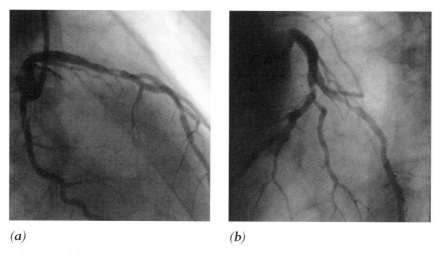

(a)   *(b)*

Figure 24.2. *Coronary angiograms 1 day later than in Fig. 24.1 after treatment with abciximab; (**a**) RAO and (**b**) LAO. The angiograms show an eccentric, circumscribed lesion proximal to the origin of D1.*

The current case demonstrates the effectiveness of abciximab in the lysis of intraluminal thrombus. *In vivo* studies have demonstrated that glycoprotein IIb/IIIa inhibition adjunctive to fibrinolytic therapy accelerates reperfusion and prevents reocclusion in canine models of coronary

128

thrombosis.[4–6] Additional observations from both animals and humans suggest that glycoprotein IIb/IIIa inhibition in the absence of exogenously applied plasminogen activators promotes coronary reflow.[7] In the literature there are several case reports that describe a thrombolytic effect of abciximab on intraluminal thrombus.[8–9]

In this case, pretreatment with abciximab resulted in the resolution of the intravascular thrombus and the uncovering of the underlying atherosclerotic plaque. In addition, it demonstrated that there was no additional disease in the diagonal branch, which led to a change in the planned procedure. This case might support a pretreatment strategy with glycoprotein IIb/IIIa inhibitors in patients with intraluminal thrombus before intervention in order to uncover the underlying disease and to reduce the risk of the subsequent intervention.

References

1. Randomised placebo-controlled trial of abciximab before and during coronary intervention in refractory unstable angina: the CAPTURE Study. *Lancet* 1997; **349**:1429–35.

2. Platelet Receptor Inhibition in Ischemic Syndrome Management in Patients Limited by Unstable Signs and Symptoms (PRISM-PLUS) Study Investigators. Inhibition of the platelet glycoprotein IIb/IIIa receptor with tirofiban in unstable angina and non-Q-wave myocardial infarction. *N Engl J Med* 1998; **338**:1488–97.

3. Hayes R, Chesebro JH, Fuster V et al. Antithrombotic effects of abciximab. *Am J Cardiol* 2000; **85**:116–72.

4. Gold HK, Coller BS, Yasuda T et al. Rapid and sustained coronary artery recanalization with combined bolus injection of recombinant tissue-type plasminogen activator and monoclonal antiplatelet GPIIb/IIIa antibody in a canine preparation. *Circulation* 1988; **77**:670–7.

5. Collet JP, Montalescot G, Lesty C et al. Disaggregation of *in vitro* preformed platelet-rich clots by abciximab increases fibrin exposure and promotes fibrinolysis. *Arterioscler Thromb Vasc Biol* 2001; **21**:142–8.

6. Yasuda T, Gold HK, Fallon JT et al. Monoclonal antibody against the platelet glycoprotein (GP) IIb/IIIa receptor prevents coronary artery reocclusion after reperfusion with recombinant tissue-type plasminogen activator in dogs. *J Clin Invest* 1988; **81**:1284–91.

7. Gold HK, Garabedian HD, Dinsmore RE et al. Restoration of coronary flow in myocardial infarction by intravenous chimeric 7E3 antibody without exogenous plasminogen activators. Observations in animals and humans. *Circulation* 1997; **95**:1755–9.

8. Ammann P, Naegeli B, Schuiki E, Bertel O. [Lysis of an intracoronary thrombus with a glycoprotein IIb/IIIa antagonist]. *Schweiz Med Wochenschr* 2000; **130**:336.

9. Russo G, Nicosia A, Tamburino C et al. [Dissolution of acute stent thrombosis by abciximab bolus]. *Cardiologia* 1998; **43**:631–4.

Case 25

NO-REFLOW AFTER BALLOON ANGIOPLASTY FOR FAILED THROMBOLYSIS IN ACUTE MYOCARDIAL INFARCTION

Stefan Verheye

Background

A 72-year-old male with no relevant medical history was admitted to a community hospital because of severe and sudden-onset chest pain. The electrocardiogram (ECG) showed marked ST elevations in the precordial leads, and the diagnosis of an acute and extensive anterior wall myocardial infarction was made. Approximately 60 minutes after the pain had started the patient received a bolus of rtPA followed by a continuous infusion. He also received aspirin IV as well as nitroglycerin and heparin. There were no electrocardiographic signs of reperfusion and 3.5 hours after the onset of pain, the patient developed sustained ventricular tachycardia and ventricular fibrillation. He was resuscitated successfully and transfer to a tertiary center was organized. On admission to our hospital, the patient was alert, hypotensive (80/50 mmHg) and the ECG showed a sinus tachycardia with marked ST elevation. He was immediately transferred to the catheterization laboratory where a diagnostic coronary angiography was performed 4.5 hours after the onset of symptoms.

Angiographic commentary

Since it was an anterior wall myocardial infarction, the right coronary artery (RCA) was injected first; it showed some atherosclerotic disease without angiographic-significant stenoses. Angiographic visible collaterals were absent (Fig. 25.1).

The left coronary artery (LCA) showed an occlusion of the left anterior descending (LAD) artery just distal to the first diagonal branch (D1). The circumflex (Cx) artery was diffusely diseased with a tight stenosis in its

131

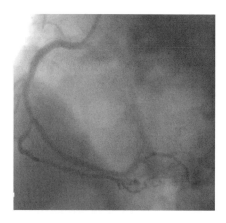

Figure 25.1. *Angiogram of the RCA showing some mild atherosclerotic disease without significant stenoses. Collaterals to the LAD cannot be seen.*

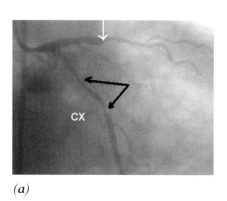

(a)

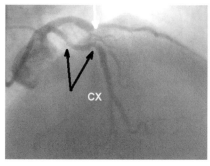

(b)

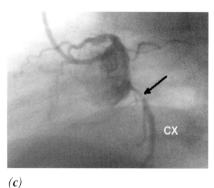

(c)

Figure 25.2(a–c). *Angiogram at the start of the procedure showing the occlusion of the mid-LAD (white arrow), and the stenosis and thrombus in the Cx (black arrows).*

proximal segment and a contrast filling defect distal to the stenosis. Based on the history of the patient, it was considered to be thrombus (Figs. 25.2a–c). Again, collaterals from the Cx to the LAD were absent.

Considering the acute infarction (ongoing ST elevation) and the unstable hemodynamic condition, despite thrombolytic therapy, it was decided to try

132

disobliteration of the LAD occlusion followed by balloon angioplasty and stenting. The LAD was easily wired and a balloon was inflated with no balloon indentation left (3.0 mm diameter, 20 mm long balloon at 8 atmospheres) at the occlusive site (Figs 25.3a and b). However, after balloon deflation and withdrawal of the balloon into the guiding catheter, there was no filling of the LAD during contrast injection (Fig. 25.4). It was decided to redilate and to administer glycoprotein IIb/IIIa receptor inhibitors IV (despite the thrombolytic treatment), as well as adenosine (4 mg in 2 ml saline) and nitrates, intracoronary, to overcome this no-reflow phenomenon. At this time, the situation became worse: there was clear visualization of a big thrombus-like filling defect in the Cx with TIMI grade 2 flow and the arterial pressure dropped. Therefore, the Cx was wired and dilated (3.0 mm diameter, 20 mm long balloon) at its obstructive site (Figs 25.5a and b). Yet, there was no-reflow (Fig. 25.6) in the Cx and a stent (3.0 mm diameter, 23 mm long at 12 atmospheres) was implanted (Fig. 25.7). In spite of these actions, the situation remained critical due to no-reflow in the LAD and no-reflow in the Cx. The arterial systolic pressure dropped to 40 mmHg, despite plasma expanders and vasopressors, and the patient developed bradycardia, became cyanotic and was dying (Fig. 25.8). High doses of intracoronary adenosine were administered but the situation did not improve acutely. Despite many attempts, it was decided to stop the intervention and not to intervene with an intraaortic balloon pump.

Surprisingly, after removing the wires and the guiding catheter from the patient, arterial pressure increased gradually, the patient started to breathe normally again, and became less pale and alert.

The guiding catheter was again introduced and positioned in the ostium of the left main artery. Contrast injection showed that there was TIMI grade 3 flow in the Cx (with a residual lesion proximally) and partial filling of the LAD (TIMI grade 1 flow (Figs 25.9a and b). Administration of nitrates and adenosine further improved the angiographic result (Fig. 25.10). Both coronary arteries were wired again and a stent (3.5 mm diameter, 28 mm long at 10 atmospheres) was implanted in the mid-LAD (Fig. 25.11). Distal from the stent, a thrombus-like filling defect within the LAD was observed (Fig. 25.12). Shortly thereafter, the patient developed ventricular tachycardia that turned into ventricular fibrillation; the patient was defibrillated successfully. Again, adenosine and nitrates were given at high doses intracoronary, and the flow in the LAD improved. The filling defect in the mid-part of the LAD had disappeared. Because of a residual stenosis in the proximal part of the Cx, just proximal to the stent, a second short stent (3.0 mm diameter, 13 mm long at 12 atmospheres) in the Cx was successfully implanted (Fig. 25.13). A final angiogram of the LCA was taken

133

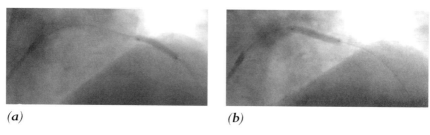

(a)   *(b)*

Figure 25.3(a and b). *Position of the angioplasty balloon in the mid-LAD.*

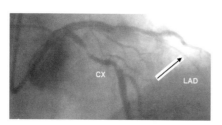

Figure 25.4. *Absence of flow in the LAD after angioplasty of the LAD (arrow is showing the wire in the LAD).*

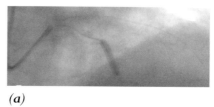

(a)

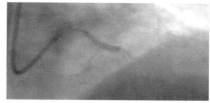

(b)

Figure 25.5(a and b). *Position of the angioplasty balloon in the Cx.*

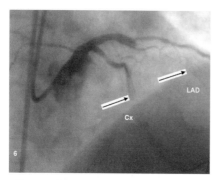

Figure 25.6. *Absence of flow in both the LAD and the Cx after angioplasty of the Cx (arrows indicate no-reflow in the LAD and the Cx).*

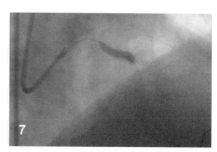

Figure 25.7. *Position of the stent implantation in the Cx.*

134

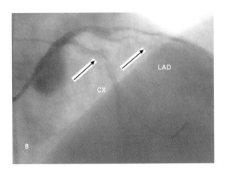

Figure 25.8. *Angiogram showing absence of flow in both vessels at the time when it was decided to stop further intervention.*

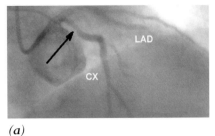

(a)

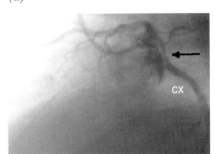

(b)

Figure 25.9 (a and b). *Contrast injection showing TIMI flow 3 in the Cx and TIMI grade 1 flow in the LAD. The black arrow indicates the presence of a residual stenosis proximal to the stent in the Cx.*

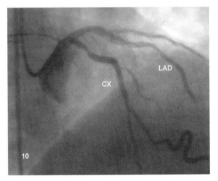

Figure 25.10. *Administration of adenosine and nitrates further improves the angiographic result.*

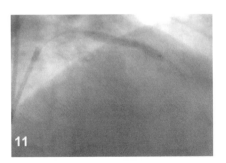

Figure 25.11. *Position of the stent implantation in the LAD.*

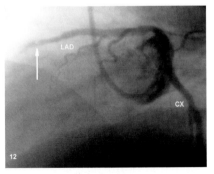

Figure 25.12. *LAO (90°) view shows good filling of the Cx and partial filling of the LAD with the presence of a filling defect in the mid-LAD (white arrow).*

135

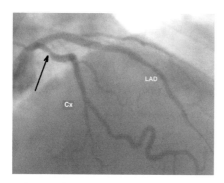 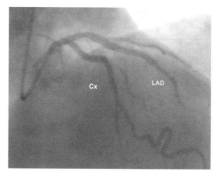

Figure 25.13. *Angiographic result just prior to implantation of a second stent in the proximal part of the Cx (black arrow).*

Figure 25.14. *Final angiogram showing distal filling of the Cx and incomplete filling of the LAD.*

and showed that both vessels were patent with TIMI grade 3 flow in the Cx and TIMI grade 1–2 flow in the LAD (Fig. 25.14).

At the end of the procedure, the patient was doing relatively well, both clinically and hemodynamically. He was transferred to the coronary care unit and discharged from the hospital 4 weeks after his acute coronary event. The transthoracic echocardiogram performed before discharge showed the presence of a large akinetic anterior wall.

Yet another patient added to the list of heart failure patients…

Discussion

This remarkable story happened whilst almost everybody else was asleep. Needless to say, during the night the operator is a single operator and, considering Murphy's Law, tough cases frequently come at that particular moment (also when thrombolytic therapy for treatment of acute infarction has failed).

Percutaneous intervention of an AMI is always challenging, since as an operator one cannot predict what exactly will occur. Realizing that thrombolysis has failed, as well as noticing the absence of collateral flow to the LAD in the presence of an acute anterior infarction, one concludes that speed is the message, since time is muscle.

At first glance, tackling the LAD looked straightforward and was not expected to be difficult. Indeed, the wire could be placed quickly in the distal part of the vessel without any problem. At least, one hoped to be in the vessel, since there was no flow in the mid- and distal part of the LAD after having crossed the occlusion. Soon, the observation of no-reflow was confirmed after deflating the angioplasty balloon.

The no-reflow phenomenon is still a vexing problem in interventional cardiology, but fortunately does not occur very often, at least not in elective percutaneous revascularization procedures. It was described for the first time in dog coronary arteries in 1974[1] and was defined as the inability to reperfuse myocardial tissue after the removal of a coronary artery occlusion. Kloner[2] postulated that no-reflow is caused by microvascular injury within areas of the dead myocardial cells, and that it could be one form of reperfusion injury that might be observed after reperfusion of the area of reversibly and irreversibly injured myocardial cells at the end of an ischemic period.[3] In addition, Morishima et al[4] have reported that no-reflow is not only a result of injury to the endothelium and the myocytes, but it may also lead to further damage of the vasculature after reperfusion. Furthermore, many reports have described the increased capillary resistance in the no-reflow area. It therefore seems obvious that no-reflow is found on the coronary angiogram as a delayed entrance of dye into the vessels that is also found to be reversible, as illustrated in this case.

The likelihood of no-reflow in this particular case was very high and could have been predicted. This is based on two reasons: firstly, there was a persistent high ST elevation after thrombolysis and before angioplasty, which has been found to be associated with a worse outcome and an increased chance of no-reflow; secondly, as described by Jeremy et al,[5] collateral coronary flow and the duration of ischemia are inversely related to the extent of the no-reflow region, at least in experimental settings.

Attempts to prevent reperfusion damage have been of limited efficacy and protection of the ischemic myocardium from this kind of injury remains unsolved. Recent reports on the administration of specific anti-CD 18 monoclonal antibodies to limit the infarct size have been disappointing.[6] On the other hand, adenosine (intracoronary or IV) has been found to positively influence no-reflow and thus the infarct size.[7–9] As illustrated in this case, it appears that not only disobliteration by angioplasty but also intracoronary administration of high doses of adenosine (and possibly glycoprotein IIb/IIIa receptor inhibitors) and nitrates may have reversed the acute critical situation, and therefore saved the life of this patient.

However, there still remain a lot of open issues. What exactly is the role of glycoprotein IIb/IIIa receptor blockers in combination with thrombolytic agents and balloon angioplasty in this setting? Secondly, would it have been possible to avoid the critical situation by not dilating the Cx artery and tackling the LAD only? Thirdly, would initial placement of an intraaortic

137

balloon pump (or use of a distal protection device), have altered the procedural outcome? And finally, should we still consider thrombolytic treatment as first choice in acute anterior wall myocardial infarction?

References

1. Kloner RA, Ganote CE, Jennings RB. The 'no-reflow' phenomenon after temporary coronary occlusion in the dog. *J Clin Invest* 1974; **54**:1496–508.

2. Kloner RA. No-reflow revisited. *J Am Coll Cardiol* 1989; **14**:1814–15.

3. Kloner RA. Does reperfusion injury exist in humans? *J Am Coll Cardiol* 1993; **21**:537–45.

4. Morishima I, Sone T, Mokuno S et al. Clinical significance of no-reflow phenomenon observed on angiography after successful treatment of acute myocardial infarction with percutaneous transluminal coronary angioplasty. *Am Heart J* 1995; **130**:239–43.

5. Jeremy RW, Links JM, Becker LC. Progressive failure of coronary flow during reperfusion of myocardial infarction: documentation of the no reflow phenomenon with positron emission tomography. *J Am Coll Cardiol* 1990; **16**:695–704.

6. Baran KW. Limitation of myocardial injury following thrombolysis in acute myocardial infarction (LIMIT). An angiographic safety and efficacy trial of a novel anti-CD 18 therapy in acute myocardial infarction in conjunction with thrombolysis. European Society of Cardiology, Amsterdam 2000.

7. Marzilli M, Orsini E, Maraccini P, Testa R. Beneficial effects of intracoronary adenosine as an adjunct to primary angioplasty in acute myocardial infarction. *Circulation* 2000; **101**:2154–9.

8. Nichols WW, Nicolini FA, Yang BC et al. Adenosine protects against attenuation of flow reserve and myocardial function after coronary occlusion and reperfusion. *Am Heart J* 1994; **127**:1201–11.

9. Pitarys CJ, Virmani R, Vildibill Jr HD et al. Reduction of myocardial reperfusion injury by intravenous adenosine administered during the early reperfusion period. *Circulation* 1991; **83**:237–47.

Case 26

Closure Of A Coronary Artery Fistula Using A Polytetrafluoro-ethylene (PTFE)-Covered Stent

Elliot Smith and Nicholas Curzen

Case history

A 55-year-old female with insulin-dependent diabetes and hypercholesterolaemia, presented to her local cardiologist with classical exertional angina. A conventional exercise test was equivocal and her tolerance of the treadmill was unsatisfactory. Angiography showed a fistula from the proximal left anterior descending (LAD) artery to the pulmonary artery (Figs 26.1–26.3). There was a considerable step down in size from the LAD up to the origin of the fistula and beyond, where there was some atheroma. The other coronaries contained minor atheromatous irregularities only. Left ventricular (LV) function was good.

This patient was referred for consideration of closure of the fistula. A thallium scan was requested and demonstrated reversible anterior wall ischaemia. The clinical impression was therefore that the angina was, at least to some extent, due to steal of blood from the LAD via the fistula. The following management options were then considered:

- Surgical closure of the fistula ± a left internal mammary artery (LIMA) graft to the LAD. This option was discussed with a surgeon who felt that such an operation may prove difficult and perhaps ineffective, both in terms of identifying and accessing the fistula and because of the well-established risk of recurrence following apparently successful surgery.[1]
- Coil embolization of the fistula. This was dismissed because of: (a) uncertainty that the fistula was arising from only one ostium of the LAD; and (b) because it was felt that it may prove impossible to access the fistula easily without risking LAD flow.
- Occlusion of the fistula origin(s) by the deployment of a covered stent. This was chosen as the best option because it would allow coverage of more than one fistula origin simultaneously.

Procedure

Via a Judkins left 3.5 8 French (Fr) guiding catheter, a 0.014 inch high torque floppy wire was passed into the fistula in order to help ascertain the exact point of its origin. The wire was then removed from the fistula and passed into the distal LAD. A 3.0 × 16 mm JoMed covered stent was positioned across the origin of the fistula, aiming to land the distal end within the wider part of the LAD. After the original deployment at 10 atmospheres the proximal part of the stent looked underdeployed and the flow in the fistula, whilst significantly reduced, was still clearly present (Fig. 26.4). The stent was therefore post-inflated to 16 atmospheres using a 4.5 mm non-compliant balloon. Flow was then almost completely eliminated in the fistula (Figs 26.5–26.7).

There remained an obvious step down in size in the LAD off the end of the stent but no further intervention was undertaken. The hope was that flow would gradually increase down the LAD having eliminated fistula flow.

Clinical course

The patient was reviewed at 4 months, when her angina was much improved although still present. Her exercise tolerance was such that no further intervention was contemplated.

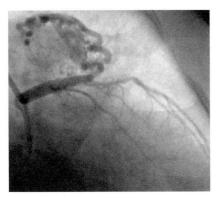

Figure 26.1. *Left coronary angiogram in right anterior oblique (RAO) projection showing fistula pretreatment. The step down in size and the diffusely diseased nature of the LAD can also be seen.*

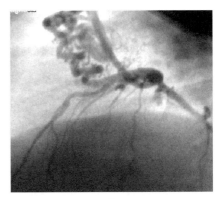

Figure 26.2. *Left coronary angiogram in left lateral projection showing fistula pretreatment.*

140

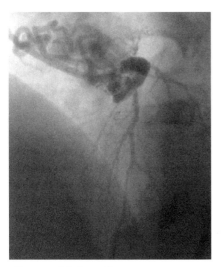

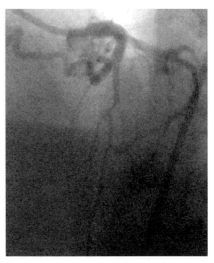

Figure 26.3. Left coronary angiogram in left anterior oblique (LAO) cranial projection showing fistula pretreatment.

Figure 26.4. Left coronary angiogram in LAO projection following initial deployment of JoMed 3 × 16 mm stent across the fistula origin to 10 atmospheres. Fistula flow is clearly reduced but still persists.

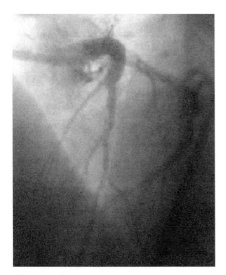

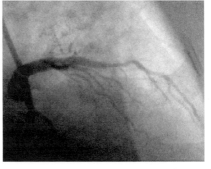

Figure 26.5. Left coronary angiogram in LAO projection following postdilation of the stent with a 4.5 × 9 mm non-compliant balloon to high pressure. Flow is now almost completely eliminated in the fistula.

Figure 26.6. Post-procedure angiogram in RAO projection.

141

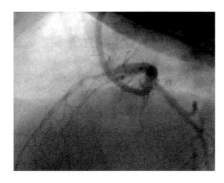

Figure 26.7. *Post-procedure angiogram in left lateral projection.*

Commentary

The JoMed stent graft is a stent device covered with a PTFE membrane. The covered stent has been described as of value to the interventionalist in a variety of settings:[2] vein graft disease;[3] ostial lesions; coronary rupture with or without aneurysm;[4] restenosis;[5] occlusion of fistulae.

This case demonstrates the value of the covered stent in the latter setting. Restenosis rates may be lower for these devices, which is clearly of critical importance in this type of case when the vessel in which the stent is deployed has the role of 'innocent bystander'. How this technique compares to embolization of the fistula itself remains contentious. It has, however, clearly expanded the armoury of the interventionalist in this setting.

References

1. Curzen NP, Gerlis L, Somerville J. A rare coronary artery to left ventricular fistula: a surgical saga. *Br J Cardiol* 1995; **2**:176–9.

2. Baldus S, Koster R, Elsner M et al. Treatment of aorto-coronary vein graft lesions with membrane-covered stents: a multicentre surveillance trial. *Circulation* 2000; **102**:2024–7.

3. Columbo A, Tobis J. A comparison of current stents. In: *Techniques in Coronary Artery Stenting.* (Martin Dunitz: London, 2000) Chapter 2.

4. Elsner M, Auch-Schwelk W, Britten M et al. Coronary stent grafts covered by a PTFE membrane. *Am J Cardiol* 1999; **84**:335–8 (abstract 8).

5. Elsner M, Britten M, Auch-Schwelk W et al. Distribution of neointimal proliferation in human coronary arteries treated with PTFE stent grafts. *J Am Coll Cardiol* 1999; **33**:17A (abstract).

Case 27

Catheter Closure Of A Large Atrial Septal Defect (ASD) Using The Amplatzer Septal Occluder (ASO) Device

Ziyad M Hijazi and Qi-Ling Cao

Background

A 67-year-old male patient was diagnosed by his referring physician as having a large secundum ASD with enlarged right atrium and ventricle (RVED dimension 40 mm). He had dyspnea on exertion and was easily fatigued. He was referred for the possibility of catheter closure using the Amplatzer septal occluder (ASO) device.

The patient's physical examination was remarkable for a prominent right ventricle impulse, normal first heart sound, grade II–VI systolic ejection murmur (heard best at the left upper sternal border), fixed splitting of the second heart sound and a diastolic rumble. An electrocardiogram (ECG) revealed a normal sinus rhythm, intraventricular conduction delay and rsR′ in V3R. A chest X-ray revealed an enlarged heart with increased pulmonary vascular markings.

After an informed consent was obtained, the patient underwent routine right and left heart catheterization with the intention of closing the defect with a device. The Qp/Qs ratio was 3:1. Transesophageal echocardiogram (TEE) under general endotracheal anesthesia revealed the presence of large secundum ASD measuring 36 × 32 mm in the short and long axis views respectively, with an absent anterior rim and a short superior rim (Figs 27.1a and b).

Following a previously reported protocol,[1] an angiogram was performed in the right upper pulmonary vein in the left anterior oblique (LAO) view with cranial angulation (four-chamber view), which revealed the presence of a large defect (Fig. 27.2a). The balloon-stretched diameter of the defect was measured to be 38–40 mm. A 40 mm ASO device (AGA Medical Corp.,

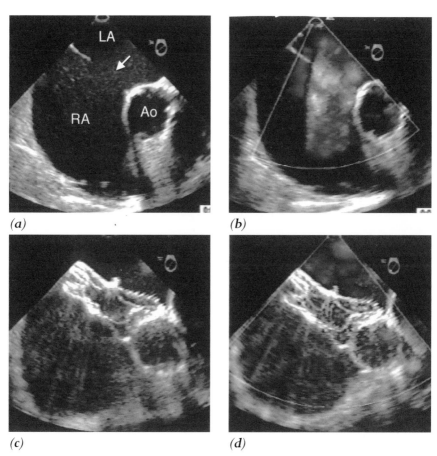

(a)   *(b)*

(c)   *(d)*

Figure 27.1. *TEE images in the short-axis view pre- (**a**, **b**) and post- (**c**, **d**) closure with the ASO device. (**a**) Without and (**b**) with color Doppler, demonstrating large secundum ASD (arrow) with the absence of the anterior rim. (**c**) Without and (**d**) with color Doppler after implantation of a 40 mm ASO device, demonstrating good device position with no residual shunt. (LA, Left atrium; RA, right atrium.)*

Figure 27.2. *(**a**) Right upper pulmonary vein angiogram in the four-chamber view demonstrating the large ASD with left-to-right shunt (arrows) (RA, right atrium; LA left atrium). (**b**) Cine image during deployment of the left atrial disc. (**c**) Cine image during deployment of the connecting waist of the device. (**d**) Angiogram through the side arm of the delivery sheath in the right atrium while the device was still attached to the delivery cable to confirm good device position. (**e**) Angiogram in the right atrium in the four-chamber view after the device had been released, demonstrating good device position. (**f**) The pulmonary levophase of the angiogram in the right atrium demonstrating no residual shunt and good device position.*

144

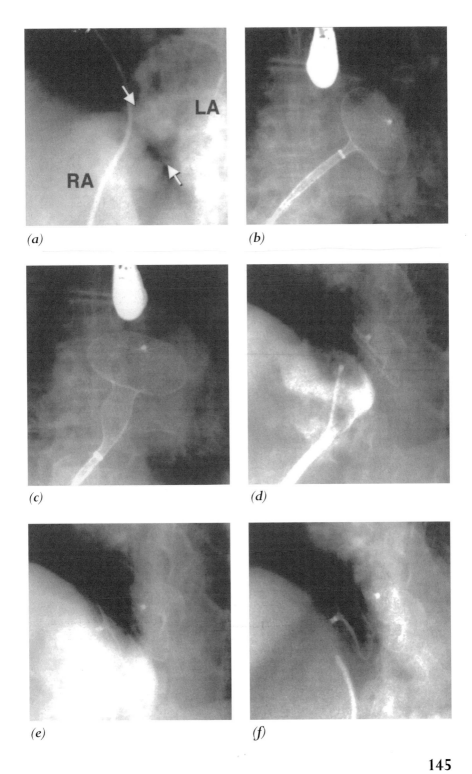

(a)

(b)

(c)

(d)

(e)

(f)

Golden Valley, MN) was successfully deployed through a 14 French (Fr) sheath across the defect (Figs 27.2 b–d), with complete closure of the defect documented by angiography (Figs 27.2e and f) and TEE (Figs 27.1c and d).

Follow-up at 1 month revealed improved symptoms and normal cardiac examination.

Commentary

Transcatheter closure of secundum ASD is easily done under TEE and fluoroscopic guidance using different investigational devices.[2,3] However, there are no cases reported in the English medical literature of closure of large secundum ASDs measuring >35 mm in a patient. This case illustrates the use of this new device (i.e. the ASO) to close a large secundum ASD, therefore extending the limits of catheter closure of secundum ASD. The main advantage of using this device is the total control and the ability to retrieve or reposition the device prior to its release from the cable. This is the first known case of catheter closure of such a large defect using the 40 mm ASO.

References

1. Masura J, Gavora P, Formanek A, Hijazi ZM. Transcatheter closure of secundum atrial septal defects using the new self-centering Amplatzer septal occluder: initial human experience. *Cathet Cardiovasc Diagn* 1997; **42**:388–93.

2. Kaulitz R, Paul T, Hausdorf G. Extending the limits of transcatheter closure of atrial septal defects with the double umbrella device (CardioSEAL). *Heart* 1998; **80**:54–9.

3. Rao PS, Sideris EB, Hausdorf G et al. International experience with secundum atrial septal defect occlusion by the buttoned device. *Am Heart J* 1994; **128**:1022–35.

146

Case 28

COMPLEX CORONARY AND SUPRAAORTIC DISEASE: UNSTABLE ANGINA DUE TO HIGH-GRADE STENOSIS OF THE LEFT SUBCLAVIAN ARTERY

Thomas A Ischinger

Background

A 60-year-old male patient with known triple-vessel coronary disease and a prior triple coronary artery bypass graft (CABG), including a left internal mammary artery (LIMA) to the left anterior descending (LAD) 9 months previously, who had not become absolutely symptom free after bypass surgery, was admitted to the hospital with unstable angina pectoris. He had been seen for angina pectoris 2 months earlier, which had been attributed to atrial fibrillation of new onset. In addition, severe arterial hypertension and obstructive pulmonary disease had been poorly controlled and were also considered reasons for chest pain complaints.

The electrocardiogram (ECG) upon admission showed new negative T-waves over V1–V4; cardiac enzymes remained negative.

Coronary angiogram

A coronary angiogram revealed 80% proximal LAD stenosis with retrograde filling of the LIMA at the LAD injection (Fig. 28.1a), a functionally occluded left circumflex (LCx) artery and an occluded right coronary artery (RCA), each with patent vein grafts. Blood pressure was 180/110 mmHg. A high-grade obstruction of the left subclavian artery was evident. Aortography and a selective angiogram of the subclavian artery confirmed c. 90% stenosis in the proximal portion of the left subclavian artery (Fig. 28.1b), just proximal to the origin of the vertebral artery. Since no other lesion could account for the anterior wall ischemia, indication for balloon dilatation and stenting was established.

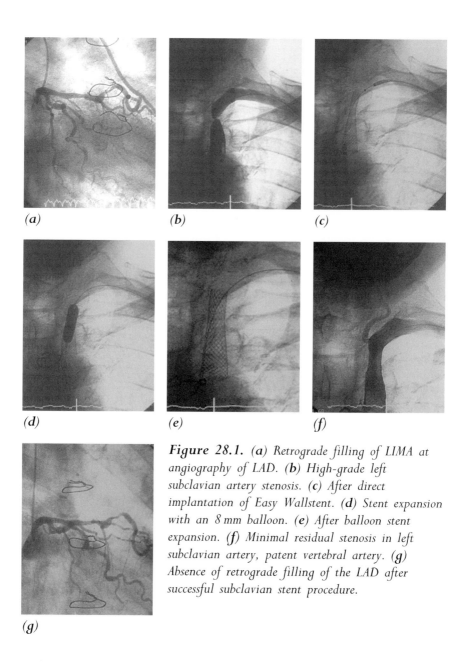

Figure 28.1. (**a**) *Retrograde filling of LIMA at angiography of LAD.* (**b**) *High-grade left subclavian artery stenosis.* (**c**) *After direct implantation of Easy Wallstent.* (**d**) *Stent expansion with an 8 mm balloon.* (**e**) *After balloon stent expansion.* (**f**) *Minimal residual stenosis in left subclavian artery, patent vertebral artery.* (**g**) *Absence of retrograde filling of the LAD after successful subclavian stent procedure.*

Procedure

A long sheath [8 French (Fr) Cook], used over a 5 Fr right coronary Judkins catheter and a 0.035 inch wire, was positioned in the ostium of the left subclavian artery. A 0.014 inch extra-support guidewire was passed through the stenosis and a 12 × 30 mm Easy Wallstent placed between the origin of the vertebral artery and the ostium of the left subclavian artery without predilatation (Fig. 28.1c). Further stent expansion was done with an 8.0 mm balloon and a residual stenosis of 25–30% was accepted (Figs 28.1d and e). Final angiography showed antegrade filling of the vertebral artery (Fig. 28.1f) and unimpaired antegrade flow into the LIMA to the LAD. Coronary angiography of the LAD confirmed flow reversal in the LIMA, since retrograde filling of the LIMA was no longer present (Fig. 28.1g).

The patient received weight-adjusted heparinization at the beginning of the procedure, and was pretreated with clopidogrel 75 mg daily and aspirin 100 mg daily. Both antiplatelet drugs were maintained for 2 months; monotherapy with clopidogrel was recommended thereafter.

Ultrasound control at 2 months revealed an excellent intermediate-term result, without progression of residual stenosis and maintenance of post-procedure flow conditions in the subclavian and vertebral artery. The patient had remained asymptomatic for myocardial ischemia.

Commentary

Since the patient had continued angina after coronary bypass surgery, we have reason to assume pre-existing subclavian disease.

The diagnosis of stenosis of the left subclavian artery was missed on probably three occasions, when its diagnosis would have been helpful. During the preoperative work-up, one would expect such vascular problems to be picked up by routine clinical and non-invasive means.

At the time of initial coronary angiography, visualization and assessment of the status of the LIMA [and the right internal mammary artery (RIMA)] is routinely performed in some centers, particularly in view of imminent coronary bypass surgery. Even though this case is anecdotal, in our experience knowledge of the condition of the LIMA and the RIMA helps in planning the surgical strategy, so visualization should be considered. In experienced hands, the risks of LIMA angiography are low, but not negligible.

At the time of surgery the subclavian stenosis was missed again and the patient was at risk of total LIMA occlusion due to competitive flow conditions.

In this case, subclavian stenting was the treatment of choice and was also recommended by the vascular surgeons. Stenting would have been the premier option prior to heart surgery too. The procedure is rewarding for the patient and can be carried out expeditiously in many instances. However,

149

knowledge about the neurovascular status of the patient and planning of the procedural strategy is needed in order not to impair cerebral flow conditions through carotid and vertebral arteries by dissection, mechanical obstruction (including bridging stents) and periprocedural embolic events.

Further reading

Diethrich EB. Initial experience with stenting in the innominate, subclavian and carotid arteries. *J Endovasc Surg* 1995; **2**:196–221.

Heuser R. In: (Beyar R, Keren G, Leon M, Serruys P, eds) *Frontiers in Interventional Cardiology: Peripheral Stenting for the Cardiologist.* (Martin Dunitz: London, 1997) 377–82.

Kumar K, Dorrios G, Bates M et al. Primary stent deployment in occlusive subclavian artery disease. *Cathet Cardiovasc Diagn* 1995; **34**:281–5.

Case 29

CATHETER-BASED CLOSURE OF A CORONARY ANEURYSM

Evelyn Regar, Chris L de Korte, Stephane G Carlier and Patrick W Serruys

Background

A 48-year-old man presented with progressive angina (CCS 3). He had a history of artery bypass grafting in 1993, and balloon angioplasty and stent implantation in the right coronary artery (RCA) in 2000 with preserved left ventricular (LV) function. His cardiovascular risk profile included hyperlipoproteinemia, hypertension and a family history of coronary artery disease. Current cardiac medication consisted of nitrates, beta-blocking agents, calcium antagonist, statin and long-term treatment with aspirin 100 mg daily.

Angiographic commentary

Biplane coronary angiography of the left coronary artery (LCA) system showed a 90% lumen diameter stenosis of the proximal left anterior descending (LAD) artery proximal to the first septal, and a large diagonal branch and a coronary aneurysm in the mid-portion of the left circumflex (LCx) artery (Fig. 29.1a).

A covered, premounted balloon-expandable stent (JoMed) with a diameter of 3.5 mm and a length of 12 mm was carefully positioned to cover the base of the aneurysm (Fig. 29.1b), and delivered at a pressure of 16 atmospheres (Fig. 29.1c). The final angiogram shows good antegrade flow (TIMI grade 3 flow) in the main lumen and complete coverage of the false lumen (Fig. 29.1d).

Intravascular ultrasound (IVUS)

IVUS provided detailed information about the vessel wall structure. The vessel showed diffuse atherosclerosis with an obstructive eccentric lesion proximal to the aneurysm (Fig. 29.2a) and eccentric low-echogenic plaque

151

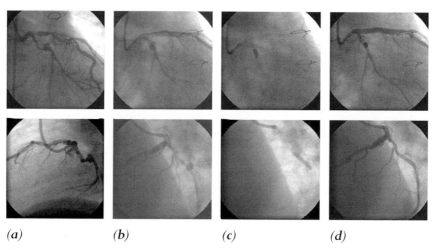

(a)   *(b)*   *(c)*   *(d)*

Figure 29.1. *Biplane coronary angiography of the left coronary artery system at* **(a)** *preintervention showing an aneurysm in the mid-portion of the left circumflex artery,* **(b)** *stent positioning (premoulded balloon-expandable covered 3.5/12 mm stent, JoMed),* **(c)** *stent implantation at 16 atmospheres and the final result* **(d)***.*

formation distally (Fig. 29.2e). Within the aneurysm, the vessel wall appeared as a single echogenic layer in its aneurysmal portion, while on the opposite side mixed fibrous–fatty plaque formation was visible. The real lumen diameter reached 3.1 mm with a total lumen area of 8.7 mm^2. Maximal extension of the false lumen reached 7.2 mm (Fig. 29.2b). A mobile echogenic structure was visible between the real and the false lumen [Fig. 29.2c (small arrows) and d]. Bolus injection of regular contrast medium indicated communication between the original vessel lumen and the aneurysmal neolumen without evidence for intraluminal thrombus formation. This was confirmed by visualization of the coronary flow in both the real and the false lumen using ChromaFlo. In this imaging mode, the IVUS echogram is combined with qualitative blood flow information (Fig. 29.3).

We interpreted this finding as an atherosclerotic pseudoaneurysm, whereby the mobile structure is an unhealed remnant of a fibrous cap after rupture of an eccentric, lipid-rich plaque, with the cavity of this plaque forming the false lumen. This hypothesis is supported by the analysis of the mechanic tissue properties using IVUS elastography.[1,2] IVUS elastography provides the local mechanical properties of the arterial wall and plaque. The color-coded elastogram (Fig. 29.4) shows relatively hard material in the suspected cap (low strain, red color) and soft material (high strain, green color) distal to it, corresponding to fibrous and fatty plaque material, respectively.

152

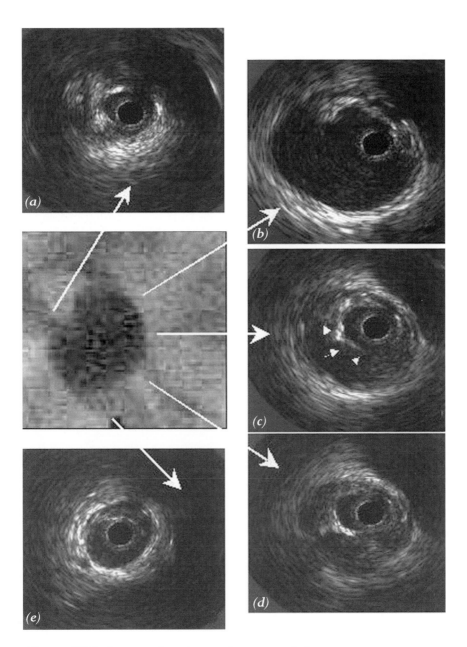

Figure 29.2. *Intravascular ultrasound imaging of the coronary aneurysm showing an eccentric plaque formation proximal* (**a**) *and distal* (**e**) *to the aneurysm. Within the aneurysm, the vessel wall appeared as a single echogenic layer on its aneursymatic portion.* (**b**) *A mobile echogenic structure was visible between the real and false lumen* (**c**, *small arrows; and* **d**).

153

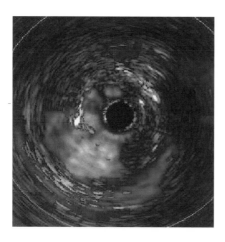

Figure 29.3. Color-coded visualization of the coronary flow with IVUS (Chromaflo™) in both, the real and false lumens.

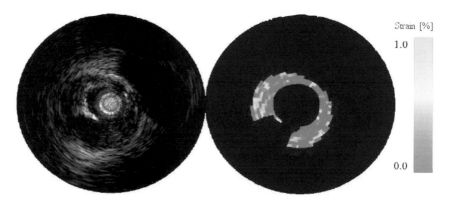

Figure 29.4. Assessment of the local mechanic properties of the arterial wall with IVUS elastography. The color-coded elastogram shows relatively hard material in the suspected ruptured plaque cap (low strain, red color) and soft material (high strain, green color) distal to it corresponding to fatty plaque material.

Commentary

Coronary artery aneurysms still remain rare findings since their early post-mortem description by Morgagni in 1761.[3] Over the past decade, they have been described with increased frequency, which might be explained by the widespread use of coronary angiography and new catheter-based treatment options. However, most of the cases are reported individually and there is a paucity of data on prognosis and controlled treatment strategies.

154

Definition and incidence

Coronary artery aneurysms are defined as a coronary dilatation that exceeds the diameter of normal adjacent segments or the diameter of the patient's largest coronary vessel by 1.5 times.[4] The incidence in angiographic series is reported to be 1.5–5%.[4–7] Pathologists distinguish between real aneurysms, characterized by ectasia of the complete vessel wall, including media and adventitia, and false or pseudoaneurysms with a disrupted artery wall.[8]

Etiology

The etiology of coronary artery aneurysms varies widely. The most important etiologic factor, accounting for c. 50% of coronary aneurysms in adults, is atherosclerosis,[5,9–11] including interventional vessel trauma,[12–15] e.g. balloon angioplasty,[16–19] cutting balloon,[20] directional coronary atherectomy,[21–23] stent implantation[24–27] and laser angioplasty.[28]

Other possible etiologies include congenital lesions,[29–31] mycotic lesions,[32–34] Kawasaki disease,[35] Marfan syndrome or Takayasu arteritis.[36] Sporadic association with systemic diseases such as syphilis, systemic lupus erythematosus,[37–40] idiopathic hypereosinophilic syndrome,[41] Behcet's disease,[42] or neurofibromatosis[43] have been described. Furthermore, chest trauma[44,45] is suggested as a possible cause of coronary aneurysm formation.

Clinical presentation

Most of the coronary aneurysms remain clinically asymptomatic. Large aneurysms may be detected sporadically in chest X-rays as a mediastinal mass.[46,47] Rare symptomatic presentations include atypical chest pain,[48] angina[49] with myocardial ischemia,[50] myocardial infarction[51–56] or sudden death.[57]

Prognosis

Little is known about the course and prognosis of aneurysmal lesions. Two major events seem to be of prognostic relevance: the rupture of the arterial aneurysm and thrombosis with possible embolization.

Aneurysm rupture is known only from pathologic series, with an incidence of 12–40%. These series included all coronary aneurysms, regardless of their etiology.[8,58] As the numbers in these series were rather small, it was not possible to identify predictors for such an event. Tunick et al[59] reported 12 patients with coronary obstructive lesions and coronary aneurysms who underwent coronary bypass surgery. In the follow-up period

155

(mean 30 months) no aneurysm rupture was seen. Similarly, no patient with a history suggestive for aneurysm rupture was seen during a follow-up period of 5 years in a series of 22 patients.[60] These data suggest that the risk of aneurysm rupture in patients with coronary artery disease is rather small.

Thrombus formation and consecutive myocardial infarction occurs more frequently in aneurysmatic coronary disease.[18,61] Analysis of the Coronary Artery Surgery Study (CASS) registry revealed that patients with aneurysms had a higher incidence of documented myocardial infarction.[4] In contrast, Demopoulos et al[62] recently reported no increased incidence (61.6 versus 64.2%) of myocardial infarction in patients with atherosclerotic aneurysms ($n = 172$) in retrospective comparison with patients with significant coronary artery disease ($n = 165$). In another series of 22 patients with atherosclerotic coronary aneurysm, two patients developed myocardial infarction during 5 years follow-up.[60] In a series with 20 patients, two cardiac deaths were observed during a mean of 30 months follow-up.[63] In another series of 17 patients with non-atherosclerotic aneurysms, all patients ($n = 5$) without antiplatelet or anticoagulant therapy experienced acute myocardial infarction (AMI).[64] Twelve of 31 patients with pure coronary ectasia had a myocardial infarction related to the aneurysmatic vessel.[62] Hill et al[17] describe the formation of coronary aneurysms 11 days to 4 months after balloon angioplasty. The aneurysms were associated with newly developed stenoses in three of five patients and a distal occlusion in one of five patients. On the other hand, spontaneous regression of iatrogenic aneurysms seems possible.[65]

Treatment

The need for treatment is controversial, the most beneficial treatment is as yet uncertain.

Conservative treatment

In a large series of 172 patients, no increased incidence of myocardial infarction, unstable angina or cardiac death in patients with atherosclerotic aneurysms under usual care was seen.[62] Similarly, others have reported cases of uneventful long-term follow-up of atherosclerotic aneurysms.[18,66] Thus, in patients with aneurysms and angiographic-apparent coronary artery disease, anticoagulation therapy seems not to be justified.

Surgery

Most authors recommend surgical intervention using different techniques such as bypass grafting resection or ligation,[10,67,68] interposition of vein graft[69] or end-to-end anastomosis[70,71] in atherosclerotic aneurysms. Patients with

156

coronary aneurysms undergoing bypass surgery have the same 5-year survival rate as patients without aneurysmal disease undergoing bypass surgery.[4]

Catheter-based treatment

Today, new techniques like coil embolization[72] or use of covered stents provide new treatment options. Currently, stents are covered by autologous veins grafts or polytetrafluoroethylene (PTFE). First clinical data suggest that the implantation of covered stents allows for elimination and subsequent thrombosis of the false lumen.[73–76] A circular-shaped lumen of an appropriate size can result in optimal flow conditions being restored.[77,78] The favorable acute results seem to be maintained during follow-up.[79,80] Thus, with this technique, the risk of neoluminal rupture may be reduced, as well as the risk of thrombosis and distal embolization, and surgical intervention may be avoided. However, covered stents have to be carefully deployed under high pressure, preferably under IVUS guidance, to avoid complications, as recently reported.[81]

In our patient recurrent angina, 7 years after bypass surgery, gave the indication for intervention. Angiography showed two lesions in the left coronary system: a significant obstruction in the LAD and the aneurysmatic lesion in the LCx. IVUS imaging suggested former plaque rupture as a possible etiologic factor. Both lesions were considered significant and highly susceptible for the patient's complaints. We decided that a catheter-based multivessel treatment was best to avoid, or postpone, re-operation, and it is preserved as a future option in this relatively young individual.

Tips and tricks for covered stent implantation

- Current available covered stents are relatively bulky, therefore:
  - back-up provided by the guiding catheter is essential
  - the use of a relatively stiff guidewire is recommended
- Predilatation might be necessary to allow for advancing the stent:
  - after predilatation, contrast injection should be performed with the deflated balloon kept in place. In case of coronary rupture, the vessel can be immediately occluded by inflating the balloon
- Covered stents are relatively rigid, therefore:
  - high-pressure balloon inflation is mandatory
  - IVUS guidance should be used to aid correct stent sizing and control of stent expansion
- Neo-endothelialization is delayed in covered stents, therefore:
  - prolonged antiplatelet therapy should be prescribed (e.g. clopidogrel for a minimum of 6 months, aspirin lifelong).

157

References

1. Ophir J, Céspedes EI, Ponnekanti H et al. Elastography: a method for imaging the elasticity in biological tissues. *Ultrasound Imag* 1991; **13**:113–34.

2. Korte CLd, Steen AFWvd, Pasterkamp G, Bom N. Intravascular ultrasound elastography: assessment and imaging of elastic properties of diseased arteries and vulnerable plaque. *Eur J Ultrasound* 1998; **7**:219–24.

3. Morgagni J. *De sedibus et causis morborum* (Venetus Tom I: Epis 27, 1761).

4. Swaye PS, Fisher LD, Litwin P et al. Aneurysmal coronary artery disease. *Circulation* 1983; **67**:134–8.

5. Daoud D, Pankin D, Tulgan H et al. Aneurysms of the coronary artery: report of ten cases and review of the literature. *Am J Cardiol* 1963; **11**:228–37.

6. Oliveros RA, Falsetti HL, Carroll RJ et al. Atherosclerotic coronary artery aneurysm. Report of five cases and review of literature. *Arch Intern Med* 1974; **134**:1072–6.

7. Aintablian A, Hamby RI, Hoffman I, Kramer RJ. Coronary ectasia: incidence and results of coronary bypass surgery. *Am Heart J* 1978; **96**:309–15.

8. Scott D. Aneurysm of the coronary arteries. *Am Heart J* 1948; **36**:403–12.

9. Anabtawi IN, de Leon JA. Arteriosclerotic aneurysms of the coronary arteries. *J Thorac Cardiovasc Surg* 1974; **68**:226–8.

10. Alford Jr WC, Stoney WS, Burrus GR et al. Recognition and operative management of patients with arteriosclerotic coronary artery aneurysms. *Ann Thorac Surg* 1976; **22**:317–21.

11. Vranckx P, Pirot L, Benit E. Giant left main coronary artery aneurysm in association with severe atherosclerotic coronary disease. *Cathet Cardiovasc Diagn* 1997; **42**:54–7.

12. Holmes Jr DR, Vlietstra RE, Mock MB et al. Angiographic changes produced by percutaneous transluminal coronary angioplasty. *Am J Cardiol* 1983; **51**:676–83.

13. Shiraishi S, Kusuhara K, Iwakura A et al. Surgical treatment of coronary artery aneurysm after percutaneous transluminal coronary angioplasty (PTCA). *J Cardiovasc Surg (Torino)* 1997; **38**:217–21.

14. Slota PA, Fischman DL, Savage MP et al. Frequency and outcome of development of coronary artery aneurysm after intracoronary stent placement and angioplasty. STRESS Trial Investigators. *Am J Cardiol* 1997; **79**:1104–6.

15. Berkalp B, Kervancioglu C, Oral D. Coronary artery aneurysm formation after balloon angioplasty and stent implantation. *Int J Cardiol* 1999; **69**:65–70.

16. Block PC, Myler RK, Stertzer S, Fallon JT. Morphology after transluminal angioplasty in human beings. *N Engl J Med* 1981; **305**:382–5.

17. Hill JA, Margolis JR, Feldman RL et al. Coronary arterial aneurysm formation after balloon angioplasty. *Am J Cardiol* 1983; **52**:261–4.

18. Smith MD, Cowley MJ, Vetrovec GW. Aneurysms of the left main coronary artery: a report of three cases and review of the literature. *Cathet Cardiovasc Diagn* 1984; **10**:583–91.

19. Schobel WA, Voelker W, Haase KK, Karsch KR. Occurrence of a saccular pseudoaneurysm formation two weeks after perforation of the left anterior descending coronary artery during balloon angioplasty in acute myocardial infarction. *Cathet Cardiovasc Intervent* 1999; **47**:341–6.

20. Bertrand OF, Mongrain R, Soualmi L et al. Development of coronary aneurysm after cutting balloon angioplasty: assessment by intracoronary ultrasound. *Cathet Cardiovasc Diagn* 1998; **44**:449–52.

21. Bell MR, Garratt KN, Bresnahan JF et al. Relation of deep arterial resection and coronary artery aneurysms after directional coronary atherectomy. *J Am Coll Cardiol* 1992; **20**:1474–81.

22. Prewitt KC, Laird JR, Cambier PA, Wortham DC. Late coronary aneurysm formation after directional atherectomy. *Am Heart J* 1993; **125**:249–51.

23. Moriuchi M, Saito S, Honye J et al. Plaque rupture as a cause of apparent coronary aneurysm formation following directional coronary atherectomy. *Cathet Cardiovasc Diagn* 1997; **41**:48–50.

24. Regar E, Klauss V, Henneke KH et al. Coronary aneurysm after bailout stent implantation: diagnosis of a false lumen with intravascular ultrasound. *Cathet Cardiovasc Diagn* 1997; **41**:407–10.

25. Nisanci Y, Coskun I, Oncul A, Umman S. Coronary artery aneurysm development after successful primary stent implantation. *Cathet Cardiovasc Diagn* 1997; **42**:420–2.

26. Yotsumoto G, Shimokawa S, Moriyama Y et al. Coronary artery aneurysm after stent implantation. *Jpn J Thorac Cardiovasc Surg* 1999; **47**:339–41.

27. Kitzis I, Kornowski R, Miller HI. Delayed development of a pseudoaneurysm in the left circumflex artery following angioplasty and stent placement, treated with intravascular ultrasound-guided stenting. *Cathet Cardiovasc Diagn* 1997; **42**:51–3.

28. Preisack MB, Voelker W, Haase KK, Karsch KR. Case report: formation of vessel aneurysm after stand alone coronary excimer laser angioplasty. *Cathet Cardiovasc Diagn* 1992; **27**:122–4.

29. Hirose H, Amano A, Yoshida S et al. Coronary artery aneurysm associated with fistula in adults: collective review and a case report. *Ann Thorac Cardiovasc Surg* 1999; **5**:258–64.

159

30. Katoh T, Zempo N, Minami Y et al. Coronary arteriovenous fistulas with giant aneurysm: two case reports. *Cardiovasc Surg* 1999; **7**:470–2.

31. Arsan S, Naseri E, Keser N. An adult case of Bland White Garland syndrome with huge right coronary aneurysm. *Ann Thorac Surg* 1999; **68**:1832–3.

32. Brasselet C, Maes D, Tassan S et al. [Extensive mycotic coronary aneurysm detected by echocardiography. Apropos of a case]. *Arch Mal Coeur Vaiss* 1999; **92**:1229–33.

33. Safi Jr J, Castelli JB, Kalil-Filho R, Mansur AJ. Cryptogenic mycotic aneurysm of the right coronary artery. *South Med J* 1999; **92**:67–8.

34. Osevala MA, Heleotis TL, DeJene BA. Successful treatment of a ruptured mycotic coronary artery aneurysm. *Ann Thorac Surg* 1999; **67**:1780–2.

35. Suzuki N, Seguchi M, Kouno C et al. Rupture of coronary aneurysm in Kawasaki disease. *Pediatr Int* 1999; **41**:318–20.

36. Suzuki H, Daida H, Tanaka M et al. Giant aneurysm of the left main coronary artery in Takayasu aortitis. *Heart* 1999; **81**:214–17.

37. Howe HS, Wong JS, Ding ZP et al. Mycotic aneurysm of a coronary artery in SLE – a rare complication of salmonella infection. *Lupus* 1997; **6**:404–7.

38. Koh HK, Yoo DH, Yoo TS et al. Coexistence of coronary aneurysms and total occlusion of coronary arteries in systemic lupus erythematosus. *Clin Exp Rheumatol* 1998; **16**:739–42.

39. Matayoshi AH, Dhond MR, Laslett LJ. Multiple coronary aneurysms in a case of systemic lupus erythematosus. *Chest* 1999; **116**:1116–18.

40. Dhond MR, Matayoshi A, Laslett L. Coronary artery aneurysms associated with systemic lupus. *Clin Cardiol* 1999; **22**:373.

41. Okinaka T, Isaka N, Nakano T. Coexistence of giant aneurysms of sinus of Valsalva and coronary artery aneurysm associated with idiopathic hypereosinophilic syndrome. *Heart* 2000; **84**:E7.

42. Srairi JE, Aouad A, Ghannam R et al. [Coronary aneurysm in Behcet's disease. Report of a case.] *Arch Mal Coeur Vaiss* 1998; **91**:1509–12.

43. Fuchi T, Ishimoto N, Kajinami T et al. A 23-year-old patient with neurofibromatosis associated with acute myocardial infarction, vasospasm and a coronary artery ectasis. *Int Med* 1997; **36**:618–23.

44. Westaby S, Drossos G, Giannopoulos N. Posttraumatic coronary artery aneurysm. *Ann Thorac Surg* 1995; **60**:712–3.

45. Wang SP, Shyong WC, Tsai JH et al. Development of posttraumatic coronary aneurysm: clinical implications. *Am Heart J* 1988; **115**:1306–7.

46. Chalasani P, Konlian D, Clements S. Paracardiac masses caused by a right coronary artery aneurysm and a saphenous vein graft aneurysm. *Clin Cardiol* 1997; **20**:79–81.

47. Channon KM, Wadsworth S, Bashir Y. Giant coronary artery aneurysm presenting as a mediastinal mass. *Am J Cardiol* 1998; **82**:1307–8 (abstract 11).

48. Yeo CK, Khalid Y. Solitary focal coronary artery aneurysm in a middle aged male with atypical chest pain. *Med J Malaysia* 1999; **54**:114–16.

49. Khan IA, Dogan OM, Vasavada BC, Sacchi TJ. Nonatherosclerotic aneurysm of the left circumflex coronary artery presenting with accelerated angina pectoris: response to medical management – a case report. *Angiology* 2000; **51**:595–8.

50. Kruger D, Stierle U, Potratz J et al. [Detection of stress-induced myocardial ischemia in isolated coronary ectasia and aneurysm (dilatative coronaropathy)]. *Z Kardiol* 1996; **85**:407–17.

51. Sharifi M, Murdock DK, Engelmeier RS et al. Simultaneous presence of a large coronary aneurysm and ectasia in a young patient with myocardial infarction – a case report. *Angiology* 1997; **48**:1001–5.

52. Otsuka M, Minami S, Hato K et al. Acute myocardial infarction caused by thrombotic occlusion of a coronary aneurysm. *Cathet Cardiovasc Diagn* 1997; **41**:423–5.

53. Straumann E, Niederhauser U, Meili C et al. Recurrent myocardial infarction caused by a giant coronary aneurysm. *Int J Cardiol* 1998; **63**:305–7.

54. von Rotz F, Niederhauser U, Straumann E et al. Myocardial infarction caused by a large coronary artery aneurysm. *Ann Thorac Surg* 2000; **69**:1568–9.

55. Meinert D, Mohammed Z. MRI of congenital coronary artery aneurysm. *Br J Radiol* 2000; **73**:322–4.

56. Hirsch GM, Casey PJ, Raza-Ahmad A et al. Thrombosed giant coronary artery aneurysm presenting as an intracardiac mass. *Ann Thorac Surg* 2000; **69**:611–13.

57. Walsh J, Siklos P, Al-Rufaie HK. Massive aneurysm of the right coronary artery causing sudden death. *Int J Cardiol* 1998; **64**:213–14.

58. Packard M, Wechsler H. Aneurysm of the coronary arteries. *Arch Intern Med* 1929; **43**:1–14.

59. Tunick PA, Slater J, Pasternack P, Kronzon I. Coronary artery aneurysms: a transesophageal echocardiographic study. *Am Heart J* 1989; **118**: 76–9.

60. Harikrishnan S, Sunder KR, Tharakan JM et al. Saccular coronary aneurysms: angiographic and clinical profile and follow-up of 22 cases. *Indian Heart J* 2000; **52**:178–82.

61. Rath S, Har-Zahav Y, Battler A et al. Fate of nonobstructive aneurysmatic coronary artery disease: angiographic and clinical follow-up report. *Am Heart J* 1985; **109**:785–91.

62. Demopoulos VP, Olympios CD, Fakiolas CN et al. The natural history of aneurysmal coronary artery disease. *Heart* 1997; **78**:136–41.

63. Tunick PA, Slater J, Kronzon I, Glassman E. Discrete atherosclerotic coronary artery aneurysms: a study of 20 patients. *J Am Coll Cardiol* 1990; **15**:279–82.

64. Wang KY, Ting CT, St John Sutton M, Chen YT. Coronary artery aneurysms: a 25-patient study. *Cathet Cardiovasc Intervent* 1999; **48**:31–8.

65. Abhyankar AD, Richmond DR, Bernstein L. Spontaneous regression of post-percutaneous transluminal coronary angioplasty aneurysm. *Int J Cardiol* 1997; **60**:233–8.

66. Desai PK, Ro JH, Pucillo A et al. Left main coronary artery aneurysm following percutaneous transluminal angioplasty: a report of a case and review of the literature. *Cathet Cardiovasc Diagn* 1992; **27**:113–16.

67. Nogaki H, Shioi K, Mase T et al. [Two cases of coronary artery aneurysm including one case of the left main coronary artery aneurysm]. *Jpn J Thorac Cardiovasc Surg* 1998; **46**:513–18.

68. Harandi S, Johnston SB, Wood RE, Roberts WC. Operative therapy of coronary arterial aneurysm. *Am J Cardiol* 1999; **83**:1290–3.

69. Firstenberg MS, Azoury F, Lytle BW, Thomas JD. Interposition vein graft for giant coronary aneurysm repair [in-process citation]. *Ann Thorac Surg* 2000; **70**:1397–8.

70. Bauer M, Redzepagic S, Weng Y, Hetzer R. Successful surgical treatment of a giant aneurysm of the right coronary artery. *Thorac Cardiovasc Surg* 1998; **46**:152–4.

71. Westaby S, Vaccari G, Katsumata T. Direct repair of giant right coronary aneurysm. *Ann Thorac Surg* 1999; **68**:1401–3.

72. Rath PC, Panigrahi NK, Agarwala MK et al. Coil embolization of a giant atherosclerotic coronary artery aneurysm. *J Invas Cardiol* 1999; **11**:559–62.

73. Gruberg L, Roguin A, Beyar R. Percutaneous closure of a coronary aneurysm with a vein-coated stent. *Cathet Cardiovasc Diagn* 1998; **43**:308–10.

74. Poli A, Lucreziotti S, Bossi I et al. [Coronary lesion with an aneurysm: their correction via angioplasty and the implantation of a coated stent]. *G Ital Cardiol* 1998; **28**:797–9.

75. Antonellis IP, Patsilinakos SP, Pamboukas CA et al. Sealing of coronary artery aneurysm by using a new stent graft. *Cathet Cardiovasc Intervent* 1999; **48**:96–9.

76. Heuser RR, Woodfield S, Lopez A. Obliteration of a coronary artery aneurysm with a PTFE-covered stent: endoluminal graft for coronary disease revisited. *Cathet Cardiovasc Intervent* 1999; **46**:113–16.

77. Di Mario C, Caprari M, Santoli C et al. Transcatheter repair of a large coronary pseudoaneurysm using ultrasound guidance and vein-covered stents. *G Ital Cardiol* 1997; **27**:701–5.

162

78. Perin EC. Autologous vein-coated stent for exclusion of a coronary artery aneurysm: case report with postimplantation intravascular ultrasound characteristics. *Tex Heart Inst J* 1999; **26**:223–5.

79. Di Mario C, Inglese L, Colombo A. Treatment of a coronary aneurysm with a new polytetrafluoethylene-coated stent: a case report. *Cathet Cardiovasc Intervent* 1999; **46**:463–5 (see comments).

80. Kolettis TM, Kyriakides ZS, Kremastinos DT. Treatment of a coronary artery aneurysm with a novel stent. *Clin Cardiol* 1999; **22**:759–61.

81. Campbell PG, Hall JA, Harcombe AA, de Belder MA. The JoMed covered stent graft for coronary artery aneurysms and acute perforation: a successful device which needs careful deployment and may not reduce restenosis. *J Invas Cardiol* 2000; **12**:272–6.

Case 30

RESOLUTION OF A LARGE CORONARY ANEURYSM BY USE OF A COVERED CORONARY STENT

Rainer Hoffmann

Background

The patient was a 76-year-old man with typical cardiac risk factors and recent onset of angina pectoris who presented for coronary angiography. Perfusion scintigraphy had been performed before coronary angiography and this demonstrated a reversible defect of the anterior wall. Angiography showed a short high-degree coronary stenosis in the left anterior descending (LAD) followed by a large coronary aneurysm and a further lumen narrowing at the outflow of the aneurysm. Bypass surgery and coronary angioplasty of the LAD were discussed as possible treatment alternatives. However, the patient decided against bypass surgery.

Angiographic commentary

A large coronary aneurysm could be visualized in the proximal part of the LAD with a high-degree stenosis directly before and behind the aneurysm (Fig. 30.1, left panel). Predilatation with a 3.0 mm balloon of 20 mm length (Adante balloon; Scimed) was performed to increase the lumen diameter and to allow subsequent stent delivery. A 16 mm long stent graft (JoStent coronary stent graft; JoMed/SitoMed; Fig. 30.2) was crimped on the balloon. Subsequently, the stent was delivered into the LAD and expanded by a 30 second inflation using 16 atmospheres maximum balloon pressure. Subsequent angiography demonstrated a smooth lumen contour with sealing of the aneurysm (Fig. 30.1, right panel). The patient was treated with clopidogrel (75 mg for 6 months) and aspirin (100 mg), and had an uneventful 6-month follow-up period.

165

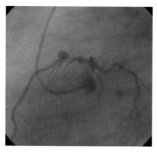 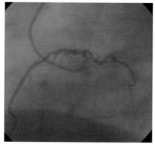

Figure 30.1. *Angiographic image of a large coronary aneurysm in the LAD before (left panel) coronary intervention and after placement (right panel) of a PTFE-covered JoStent coronary stent graft. The coronary aneurysm could be completely resolved and no stenosis remained.*

Discussion

Atherosclerotic vessel wall destruction is the most frequent underlying cause of coronary aneurysm formation, probably forming a variant of coronary atherosclerosis. Inflammatory (Kawasaki's disease) or infectious (mycotic aneurysms) illnesses are other causes. Aneurysm formation may also occur immediately after a coronary intervention, indicating a contained perforation, or late after the procedure, indicating thinning of the vessel wall. While the incidence of aneurysms may be c. 5% after balloon angioplasty, it may be as high as 10% after directional atherectomy. There is frequently a coexistence of aneurysms and stenotic lesions in close proximity. Atherosclerotic aneurysms are rarely known to rupture. However, they almost always contain thrombus. The risks of atherosclerotic aneurysms relate to possible lumen occlusion or distal embolization from the thrombotic material.

The treatment of coronary artery aneurysms for a long time comprised surgical resection and grafting. The use of conventional stents or stents covered with autologous venous material has been described as possible options to treat coronary aneurysms. Stephanadis et al[1] were the first to describe the use of vein-covered stents. Wong et al[2] described the repair of a post-atherectomy pseudoaneurysm using a Palmaz–Schatz biliary stent covered with a portion of a cephalic vein. However, harvesting of a vein is associated with additional trauma to the patient and increases the time required for the procedure.

The JoStent coronary stent graft is an elegant alternative, allowing rapid and successful treatment of a coronary aneurysm. It combines the properties of a graft and a coronary stent. It is constructed by using a sandwich technique, which includes an ultrathin layer of expandable polytetrafluoroethylene (PTFE) placed between two stents, welded as its ends. The stent construction allows

166

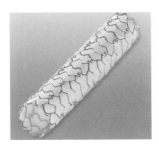

Figure 30.2. *Image of a JoStent coronary stent graft. The sandwich structure of the stent, consisting of an ultrathin layer of expandable PTFE placed between two stents, can be seen.*

sealing off of the vessel wall. It has been used effectively for coronary dissections, perforations and aneurysms.[3,4] The JoStent coronary stent graft has been expected to reduce the restenosis rate due to the prevention of intimal hyperplasia growth by the PTFE membrane. However, it proved that there is still intimal hyperplasia, which primarily affects the stent margins. Thus, lumen narrowing is pronounced at the stent margins with the overall restenosis rate not being significantly reduced compared to conventional stents.

There are some points which should be considered when using the stent graft. Delivery of the stent graft may be impeded by the relatively stiff and bulky characteristics of the sandwich construction of the stent. Stent implantation should be performed using an implantation pressure of 16 atmospheres to allow sufficient expansion of the rigid stent graft design. Side branches originating from the vessel segment to be treated by the graft stent will be occluded due to the PTFE membrane. A high rate of stent thrombosis, even several months after stent implantation, have been described with the JoStent coronary stent graft. This has been ascribed to the reduced rate of intimal hyperplasia in the body of the stent. Clopidogrel should be administered for a 6-month period to reduce the rate of stent thrombosis.

References

1. Stephanadis C, Karayannakos P, Kallikazaros I et al. Transluminal vascular stenting using autologous vein grafts. *Eur Heart J* 1992; **13**:260 (supplement).

2. Wong SC, Kent KM, Mintz GS et al. Percutaneous transcatheter repair of a coronary aneurysm using a composite autologous cephalic vein-coated Palmaz–Schatz biliary stent. *Am J Cardiol* 1995; **76**:990–1.

3. Gerckens U, Müller R, Cattelaens N et al. First clinical experiences with a covered stent: the JoStent coronary stent graft. *Int J Cardiovasc Intervent* 1998; **1**:68–74.

4. Von Birgelen C, Haude M, Liu F et al. Behandlung eines koronaren Pseudo-aneurysmas durch Stent-Graft-Implantation. *Dtsch Med Wschr* 1998; **123**:418–22.

167

Case 31

Coronary Pseudoaneurysm And A Left Anterior Descending (LAD) Artery Lesion Treated By Implantation Of A Stent Graft

Mario Gössil, Clemens von Birgelen and Raimund Erbel

Background

A 54-year-old male with hypercholesterolaemia and smoking as coronary risk factors was referred to our department with new-onset unstable angina (Braunwald class IB), characterized by accelerating new onset of chest pain with radiation in both arms but sensitive to oral nitrates. Acute myocardial infarction (AMI) was excluded by repeat electrocardiogram (ECG) and laboratory testing, including troponin I, creatine kinase (CK) and CK myocardial band (MB). Coronary angiography revealed an eccentric stenosis in the proximal LAD artery with an adjacent aneurysmatic formation distal to it. Subsequent intravascular ultrasound (IVUS) [3.2 French (Fr) 30 MHz, UltraCross; CVIS/Boston Scientific] identified the aneurysmatic formation as a coronary pseudoaneurysm due to rupture of the adjacent plaque after lipid core washout (Figs 31.1–31.3). The patient's symptoms may have resulted from thrombus formation after plaque rupture and/or additional microembolization. We decided to implant a stent graft, in order to cover both the pseudoaneurysm and the LAD stenosis, as a good therapeutic option. The coronary stent used was characterized by a polytetrafluoroethylene (PTFE) membrane fixed between two thin metal layers (90 μm each). The result after covered stent implantation is shown in Fig. 31.4.

Procedure

Via the femoral approach and a Judkins 4 8 Fr guiding catheter, a 0.014 inch floppy guidewire was positioned in the distal LAD. Because of sufficient

169

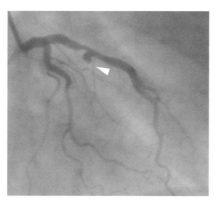

Figure 31.1. Angiogram before intervention – pseudoaneurysm and distal septal branch (white arrowhead).

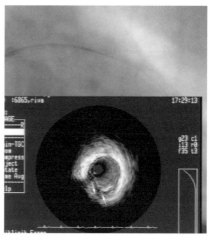

Figure 31.2. IVUS before intervention – ruptured plaque (white arrows) proximal to the pseudoaneurysm.

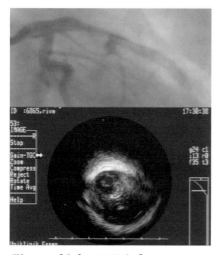

Figure 31.3. IVUS before intervention – pseudoaneurysm just distal to ruptured plaque.

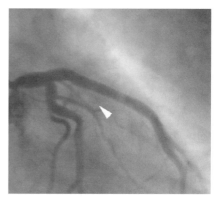

Figure 31.4. Angiogram after stent graft implantation – occluded distal septal branch (white arrowhead).

residual lumen (1.5 mm) at the site of the proximal stenosis, no predilatation was required. A 19 mm long coronary stent graft (JoStent coronary stent graft; JoMed) was mounted on a 3.5 × 20 mm balloon catheter (Maxxum; SciMed). The stent graft was implanted at 16 atmospheres to cover both the proximal lesion and the adjacent pseudoaneurysm. We could not avoid covering a distal septal branch, originating close to the pseudoaneurysm

170

(Fig. 31.5) and some dye hold-up can be seen in this small vessel. Angiographic control demonstrated that the LAD stenosis was well dilated and that the pseudoaneurysm was completely sealed. In the IVUS after stent deployment (Fig. 31.6), flow to the pseudoaneurysm was seen to be obliterated, the stent lumen was free (lumen diameter 3.0–3.6 mm) but at both stent graft extremities underdilatation was present. Accordingly, we performed postdilatation with a 4.0 × 20 mm Maxxum balloon catheter at 12 atmospheres. Angiographic control revealed a smoother transition at the graft extremities of the stent with a luminal diameter of 3.3–4.0 mm. IVUS control confirmed a smooth transition between the stent graft and the adjacent reference segments.

Clinical course

The unavoidable occlusion of an adjacent distal septal branch led to a mild asymptomatic rise of CK (maximum 173 IU/l). The patient was reviewed at 10, 16 and 28 months without any change in the ECG. There was a mild formation of neointima, particularly at the stent graft extremities.

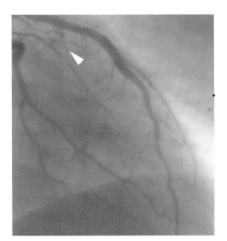

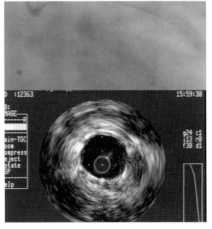

Figure 31.5. *Angiogram at 28 months follow-up — mild neointima formation and reperfusion of the initially occluded distal septal branch.*

Figure 31.6. *IVUS at 28 months follow-up — flow between the outside of the distal stent graft and the surrounding vessel wall is clearly demonstrated. In addition, the initially occluded distal septal branch was now reperfused and showed good antegrade flow.*

171

Interestingly, angiography and IVUS at follow-up clearly demonstrated flow between the outside of the distal stent graft and the surrounding vessel wall. In addition, the initially occluded distal septal branch was now reperfused and showed a good antegrade flow. At all controls, angiography and IVUS showed no significant progress of neointima formation and/or atherosclerosis, as well as no decrease in the coronary flow reserve (CFR).

Commentary

Pseudoaneurysms, which have an inherent risk of coronary rupture, can be treated by conventional stenting (CS). However, this approach implies the danger of distal embolization of thrombotic material from the plaque ulcer. In the present case we decided to seal the pseudoaneurysm by implanting a coronary stent graft covering both the adjacent proximal stenosis and the pseudoaneurysm. Sealing prevented potential embolization of thrombotic material and rupture of the pseudoaneurysm.

Side branches at the site of stent graft implantation can be critical. The unavoidable occlusion of an adjacent distal septal branch led to a mild asymptomatic rise in CK (maximum 173 IU/l. At 10 months follow-up, this branch was reperfused and there was flow between the outside of the distal stent graft and the surrounding vessel wall. Reperfusion of the septal branch may have occurred soon after the procedure, preventing thrombus formation and total occlusion of the branch. Flow between the outside of the distal stent graft and the surrounding vessel wall may be avoided by a higher balloon pressure or a higher balloon-to-artery ratio.

Our group has recently demonstrated that adequate expansion of stent grafts can only be achieved by using relatively large low-compliant balloon catheters at high pressures.[1] Recently, Campbell et al[2] suggested the use of high-pressure deployment, IVUS control and prolonged antiplatelet therapy, based on their own experience in aneurysmic and perforated coronary arteries. Follow-up data of the coronary stent graft in 40 patients showed unfavourable long-term results,[3] which has led to a suggestion to continue prolonged antiplatelet therapy with clopidogrel. Accordingly, we currently recommend 6 to 12 months of clopidogrel therapy (75 mg daily after an initial loading dose of 300 mg) in addition to lifelong aspirin therapy (100 mg daily).[4]

Although coronary stent grafts have been used successfully in several settings like coronary perforation and pseudoaneurysm,[5-8] unrestricted use should definitively be avoided.[4] So far, long-term data are equivocal concerning delayed stent thrombosis, possible perforation of the PTFE membrane, occlusion and restenosis.[4,9-11]

References

1. von Birgelen C, Haude M, Herrmann J et al. Early clinical experience with the implantation of a novel synthetic coronary stent-graft. *Cathet Cardiovasc Intervent* 1999; **47**:496–503.

2. Campbell PG, Hall JA, Harcombe AA, de Belder MA. The JoMed covered stent graft for coronary artery aneurysms and acute perforation: a successful device which needs careful deployment and may not reduce restenosis. *J Invasive Cardiol* 2000; **12**:272–6.

3. Elsner M, Auch-Schwelk W, Britten M et al. Coronary stent grafts covered by a polytetrafluoroethylene membrane. *Am J Cardiol* 1999; **84**:335–8.

4. von Birgelen C, Haude M, Erbel R. A word of caution on unrestricted use of synthetic stent grafts in native coronary arteries. *Cathet Cardiovasc Intervent* 2000; **50**:266–7.

5. von Birgelen C, Haude M, Liu F et al. Treatment of coronary pseudoaneurysm by stent-graft implantation. *Dtsch Med Wschr* 1998; **123**:418–22.

6. Welge D, Haude M, von Birgelen C et al. Management of coronary perforation after percutaneous balloon angioplasty with a new membrane stent. *Z Kardiol* 1998; **87**:948–53.

7. Di Mario C, Inglese L, Colombo A. Treatment of a coronary aneurysm with a new polytetrafluoroethylene-coated stent: a case report. *Cathet Cardiovasc Intervent* 1999; **46**:463–5.

8. Heuser RR, Woodfield S, Lopez A. Obliteration of a coronary artery aneurysm with a PTFE-covered stent: endoluminal graft for coronary disease revisited. *Cathet Cardiovasc Intervent* 1999; **46**:113–16.

9. Lukito G, Vandergoten P, Jaspers L et al. Six months clinical, angiographic, and IVUS follow-up after PTFE graft stent implantation in native coronary arteries. *Acta Cardiol* 2000; **55**:255–60.

10. Leung AW, Wong P, Wu CW et al. Left main coronary artery aneurysm: sealing by stent graft and long-term follow-up. *Cathet Cardiovasc Intervent* 2000; **51**:205–9.

11. Bosmans JM, Claeys MJ, Dilling D, Vrints CJ. Unsuccessful long-term outcome after treatment of a vein graft false aneurysm with a polytetrafluoethylene-coated JoStent. *Cathet Cardiovasc Intervent* 2000; **50**:105–8.

173

Case 32

OCCLUSION OF A CORONARY FISTULA

Philip Urban, Pierre-Alain Schneider, Patrick Schopfer and Antoine Bloch

Background

The patient was a 35-year-old female known to have had a heart murmur since the age of 13. At the age of 34, echocardiography documented an important fistula between the right coronary artery (RCA) and the right atrium: the patient remained asymptomatic. The murmur was continuous, of moderate intensity and loudest in the second right intercostal space. In August 1999, at the age of 35, a cardiac catheterization was undertaken, and revealed a pulmonary-to-systemic flow ratio (Qp/Qs) of 1.7, with mildly raised pulmonary artery pressures (30/16 mmHg). Angiography showed normal coronary anatomy, together with a very large fistula, originating in the immediate vicinity of the right coronary ostium [Fig. 32.1 – right anterior oblique (RAO) projection]. Five months later, the fistula was closed percutaneously under general anesthesia.

Procedure

A 6 French (Fr) left Amplatz catheter was positioned in the aortic ostium of the fistula. A 300 cm long, 0.014 inch wire was threaded through the fistula into the right atrium and, after retrieving it through a right femoral vein access, a 6 Fr multipurpose guiding catheter was advanced over the wire retrogradely into the fistula (Fig. 32.2 – RAO projection).

With both catheters in a stable position, it was then possible to embolize three separate 15 mm coils (Cook Inc., Bloomington, IN) retrogradely into the fistula. Angiography showed the resulting occlusion when dye was injected proximally with both catheters still in position (Fig. 32.3 – RAO projection) A final injection from the arterial side showed that there was no encroachment of the coils on the right coronary ostium (Fig. 32.4 – RAO projection; Fig. 32.5 – LAO projection).

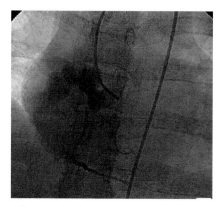

Figure 32.1.

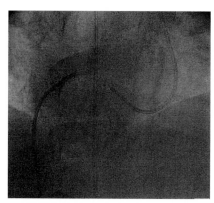

Figure 32.2.

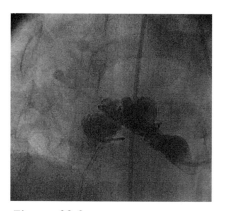

Figure 32.3.

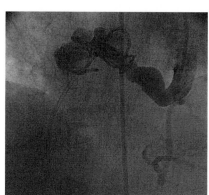

Figure 32.4.

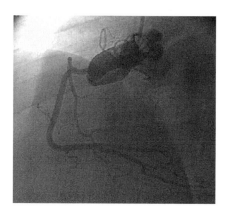

Figure 32.5.

Post-intervention course

Postoperatively, the murmur disappeared and complete closure was confirmed the next day by echocardiography. Two weeks after the intervention, the patient developed atrial fibrillation (AF). This was treated by a combination of amiodarone and warfarin. A stable sinus rhythm was restored after 2 days of treatment. The patient has now remained well and asymptomatic for >1 year; all medication was discontinued after 6 months.

Comment

Complete percutaneous closure of large coronary fistulas can generally be obtained using one or several coils. Great care must be taken so that the coils do not interfere with coronary flow; they are best positioned distally in the fistula, near the right atrial ostium. Technically, the method used in the present case has two main advantages: (a) the exchange length wire threaded from the arterial catheter through the fistula and out via the femoral vein affords excellent delivery catheter stability for precise coil positioning; (b) good angiographic visualization from both the arterial and the venous side is possible at all times during the procedure.

Reference

1. Dorros G, Thota V, Ramireddy K, Joseph G. Catheter-based techniques for closure of coronary fistulae. *Cathet Cardiovasc Intervent* 1999; **46**:143–50.

177

Percutaneous Transluminal Laser Guidewire Recanalization Of Chronic Subclavian Artery Occlusion In Symptomatic Coronary–Subclavian Steal Syndrome (CSSS)

Dietrich Baumgart, Holger Eggebrecht, Christoph K Naber, Olaf Oldenburg, Joerg Herrmann, Michael Haude and Raimund Erbel

Background

Treatment of subclavian artery stenosis by percutaneous balloon angioplasty and adjunctive stent placement has been shown to be safe and efficacious, but may be limited in tight stenoses and long occlusions. We describe a patient who developed progressive angina pectoris associated with signs of cerebrovertebral insufficiency 9 years after bypass surgery, including left internal mammary artery (LIMA) grafting to the left anterior descending (LAD) coronary artery. Angiography showed reversed flow through the LIMA graft into the subclavian artery and a 4 cm occlusion beginning at the origin of the left subclavian artery, representing a rare CSSS. After a conventional approach failed, recanalization was successfully performed using laser guidewire angioplasty with adjunctive stent placement in a combined radial and femoral approach.

Introduction

A hemodynamically significant stenosis or occlusion of the proximal left subclavian artery is a rare cause of recurrent myocardial ischemia in patients with patent LIMA grafts, resulting in coronary steal due to impaired or reversed flow through the LIMA.[1,2]

179

Percutaneous transluminal coronary angioplasty (PTCA) with adjunctive stent placement has evolved as first-line treatment of the subclavian steal and the CSSS, respectively.[3,4] However, these percutaneous techniques may be limited in tight stenoses or in the presence of chronic occlusions.[1,3]

In the present case, we describe a patient with symptomatic CSSS caused by a patent LIMA graft in the presence of an occluded left subclavian artery, which was successfully recanalized using laser guidewire angioplasty and subsequent stent implantation.

Case report

A 46-year-old male patient presented with recurrent episodes of exertional angina pectoris, occasionally even at rest [class III-IV according to the Canadian Cardiovascular Society (CCS) classification], and simultaneous occurrence of dizziness during physical exercise.

Nine years previously, the patient underwent a triple coronary artery bypass graft (CABG), including LIMA revascularization of the LAD. Stent graft placement of a saphenous vein graft (SVG) stenosis to the right coronary artery (RCA) was successfully performed 1 year before the present hospitalization, with a good long-term result.

Cardiovascular risk factors included hypertension and a family disposition to coronary artery disease (CAD). Physical examination showed a systolic blood pressure difference between the left (110/70 mmHg) and right (160/90 mmHg) arm of 50 mmHg. Arterial pulses were hardly detectable at the left radial artery. Doppler examination showed reversed flow in the vertebral artery, suggestive of a subclavian steal syndrome.

Diagnostic coronary angiography showed significant left main stem stenosis, high-grade stenosis of the mid-LAD and ostial occlusion of the RCA. Vein grafts to RCA and the left circumflex (LCx) artery were patent without significant stenosis. Strikingly, contrast injection into the left coronary artery (LCA) showed retrograde reflux through the LIMA graft into the subclavian artery without competing antegrade flow, as a characteristic sign of a CSSS (Fig. 33.1). Aortic arch angiography revealed complete occlusion of the left subclavian artery at the origin.

A recanalization attempt via the femoral approach seemed to be impossible in the absence of a vessel stump. Furthermore, the brachial approach was thwarted in the absence of palpable pulse in the left brachial artery. Therefore, left radial access was obtained by a 6 French (Fr) arterial sheath (Avanti Introducer; Cordis, Warren, USA), and 10 000 IU of heparin were administered intraarterially.

180

Simultaneous aortic arch and selective subclavian artery angiography showed an occlusion of the subclavian artery over a distance of *c.* 4.0 cm from the origin (Fig. 33.2), and simultaneous intraarterial pressure measurements showed a pressure gradient of 54 mmHg.

Subsequently, a 6 Fr Judkins right (JR) coronary guiding catheter (Super torque plus; Cordis) was advanced to the occlusion from the left radial access. An initial conventional recanalization attempt, using a hydrophilic-coated 0.014 inch guidewire (Choice PT plus; Boston Scientific, Maple Grove, USA), was not successful. Due to the long length of the occlusion, the decision was made to make a second attempt utilizing a 0.018 inch fiber-optic laser guidewire (Prima; Spectranetics Corp., Colorado Springs, USA) connected to a 308 nm xenon chloride excimer laser unit (CVX 300; Spectranetics Corp.) for recanalization. After calibration of the laser energy density, the wire was advanced to the occlusion site through a special support catheter (Spectranetics Corp.). Laser fluence was set at 60 mJ/mm^2 at a repetition rate of 25/second. After alignment of the guidewire tip with the assumed anatomic course of the subclavian artery, cautious advancement of the laser wire was monitored by fluoroscopy in different projections. After several reorientations of the wire tip, the guidewire successfully crossed the occlusion and reached access to the aorta. The intravascular position of the laser guidewire was ascertained by angiography. The laser

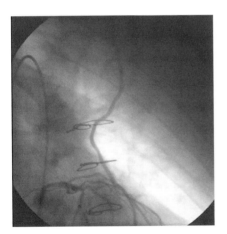

Figure 33.1. *Angiography of the LCA system showing retrograde opacification of the LIMA graft due to inversed blood flow characteristic of CSSS [right anterior oblique (30°) projection].*

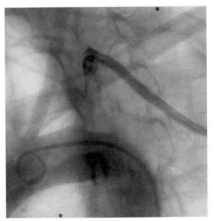

Figure 33.2. *Simultaneous angiography of the aortic arch and the left subclavian artery during laser guidewire angioplasty demonstrating the long occluded proximal vessel segment of the left subclavian artery [left anterior oblique (60°) projection].*

181

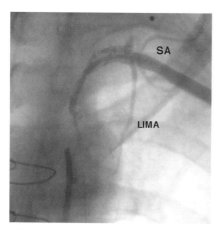 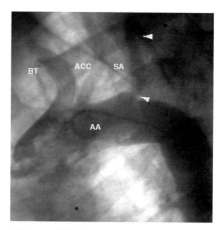

Figure 33.3. *Selective angiography after successful recanalization showing large dissection of the proximal left subclavian artery with extravasation of dye (LIMA, left internal mammary artery; SA, subclavian artery; AP, projection).*

Figure 33.4. *Post-interventional angiography of the aortic arch showing restored blood flow through the left subclavian artery [BT brachiocephalic trunk; ACC, common carotid artery; SA, subclavian artery; AA, aortic arch; arrows indicate the position of the stent; LAO (60°) projection].*

wire was exchanged for a hydrophilic-coated angioplasty guidewire (Choice PT plus; Boston Scientific) that was placed in the aortic lumen, and stepwise balloon angioplasty was performed using increasing balloon sizes from 1.5 to finally 5.0 mm. Simultaneous pressure measurement showed almost complete pressure normalization between the aorta and the subclavian artery.

Angiography revealed contrast flow from the subclavian artery to the aorta, but also a large dissection with extravasation of dye in the recanalized origin of the artery (Fig. 33.3).

Therefore, we decided to implant a stent of 7 mm in diameter and 18 mm in length (Herculink; Guidant, Temecula, USA). However, the shaft diameter of the delivery system of 6.1 Fr made an implantation via radial access impossible. Consequently, an 8 Fr JR guiding catheter (Super torque plus; Cordis) was placed in the ostium of the left subclavian artery via the femoral access. Due to the dissection, an antegrade attempt to advance a conventional 0.014 inch guidewire (ACS Hi-Torque Floppy II; Guidant) into the true lumen of the subclavian artery failed. Thus, a 7 mm Amplatz goose-neck snare (Microvena; White Bear Lake, USA) was introduced into the aorta from the radial approach via the true lumen of the subclavian artery, and the guidewire was successfully snared and pulled back into the true lumen of the subclavian artery.

182

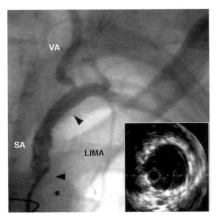

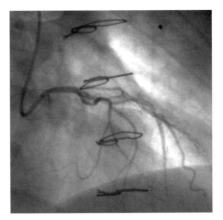

Figure 33.5. Follow-up angiography after 3 months showing a good long-term result of the recanalized left subclavian artery (SA) with antegrade perfusion of the vertebral artery (VA) and the LIMA. IVUS showed negligible neointima proliferation within the stents (AP projection).

Figure 33.6. Angiography of the LCA after recanalization of the left subclavian artery showing no retrograde opacification of the LIMA graft and competing flow in the distal LAD [RAO (30°) projection].

Subsequently, two 7.0 mm diameter by 18 mm length stents (Herculink; Guidant) were implanted via the 8 Fr JR guiding catheter from the femoral access, resulting in complete coverage of the dissection (Fig. 33.4). Final aortic arch angiography showed good contrast flow into the left subclavian artery with antegrade opacification of the LIMA graft (Fig. 33.4). Simultaneous pressure measurement showed a residual gradient of 6 mmHg. Left coronary angiography showed competing antegrade flow in the LIMA with remaining retrograde contrast reflux to the mid segment of the bypass.

Total fluoroscopy time was 37.5 minutes and the total time of laser energy delivered was 2.8 minutes.

The post-procedural course of the patient was uneventful. Clopidogrel 75 mg daily was administered for 30 days. Post-interventional Doppler examination showed antegrade perfusion of the vertebral artery. At follow-up examination after 3 months, the previously experienced symptoms of angina and dizziness on exercise had completely resolved. Control angiography revealed a good long-term result without detectable neointimal hyperplasia within the stents as assessed by intravascular ultrasound (IVUS) (Fig. 33.5). Pressure measurements showed a residual gradient of 10 mmHg. Contrast injection into the LCA showed no retrograde opacification of the LIMA graft with competing antegrade flow in the distal LAD (Fig. 33.6).

183

Discussion

Athero-occlusive disease of the aortic arch often involves the subclavian artery.[5] The left subclavian artery is affected three to four times more frequently than the right side.[6]

The incidence of CSSS due to a critical stenosis or occlusion of the subclavian artery was reported in 0.2–0.7% of patients after CABG,[1,5] and may even become more frequent with respect to the increasing utilization of LIMA grafts in surgical myocardial revascularization.

Traditional surgical treatment with carotid–subclavian bypass or subclavian–carotid transposition has been widely replaced in recent years by percutaneous techniques because of similar success rates and fewer complications.[3,7] Thus, transluminal therapy by PTCA and adjunctive stent placement has evolved as the first-line treatment for subclavian artery stenosis. Stenting of the subclavian artery was shown to improve the results of stand alone PTCA[8] with overall improved patency rates.[3] However, these techniques may be limited in recanalization of chronic total occlusions or tight stenoses.[1,4,9]

Laser energy transmitted through optical fibers has been shown to be effective in vaporizing atherosclerotic plaques and recanalizing severe or total arterial occlusions.[10] Excimer laser guidewire angioplasty has been used as a feasible and relatively safe therapeutic option for recanalization of chronic total coronary artery occlusions, refractory to treatment with mechanical guidewires.[11–13] To the best of our knowledge, so far, no experience has been reported using excimer laser guidewire angioplasty in subclavian artery occlusion.

A particular complication associated with the use of the laser guidewire is perforation of the vessel wall, since the ablative laser energy makes no distinction between vessel wall and intraluminal occlusive tissue. In coronary artery occlusion, clinical sequelae were not encountered with coronary artery perforation by the laser guidewire, probably due to the small diameter of the perforation which closed spontaneously.[11] In our patient, no extravasation of contrast was noted during the use of the laser guidewire. However, continuous monitoring of the laser guidewire by multiplane fluoroscopy and repeat realignment of the wire tip with the assumed anatomic course during recanalization is mandatory to avoid this potentially severe complication.

In our case, there were also no complications observed during the subsequent PTCA. These are rare, and may include dissection, hematoma formation or thrombosis of the vascular access site, reocclusion and distal embolization.[1,7–9] Vertebral embolic complications and subsequent stroke, with an overall incidence of c. 1%,[1] are a major concern of subclavian

PTCA. Some authors recommend temporary balloon occlusion of the vertebral artery to prevent central embolization.[14] Ringelstein and Zeumer[15] described that after subclavian angioplasty, flow reversal in the vertebral artery is delayed from 20 seconds up to several minutes, thus naturally preventing cerebellar embolization.

In conclusion, laser guidewire angioplasty provides an alternative option in the treatment of subclavian artery occlusion refractory to conventional mechanical recanalization.

References

1. Marques KM, Ernst SM, Mast et al. Percutaneous transluminal angioplasty of the left subclavian artery to prevent or treat the coronary–subclavian steal syndrome. *Am J Cardiol* 1996; **78**:687–90.

2. Kugelmass AD, Kim D, Kuntz RE et al. Endoluminal stenting of a subclavian artery stenosis to treat ischemia in the distribution of a patent left internal mammary graft. *Cathet Cardiovasc Diagn* 1994; **33**:175–7.

3. Hadjipetrou P, Cox S, Piemonte T, Eisenhauer A. Percutaneous revascularization of atherosclerotic obstruction of aortic arch vessels. *J Am Coll Cardiol* 1999; **33**:1238–45.

4. Henry M, Amor M, Henry I et al. Percutaneous transluminal angioplasty of the subclavian arteries. *J Endovasc Surg* 1999; **6**:33–41.

5. Fields WS, Lemak NA. Joint study of extracranial arterial occlusions VII. Subclavian steal: a review of 168 cases. *J Am Med Assoc* 1972; **222**:1139–43.

6. Williams SJ II. Chronic upper extremity ischemia: current concepts in management. *Surg Clin North Am* 1986; **66**:355–75.

7. Giavroglou C, Proios T, Daponte P et al. Coronary–subclavian steal syndrome: treatment with percutaneous transluminal angioplasty and stent placement. *Eur Radiol* 1999; **9**:948–50.

8. Rodriguez JA, Werner A, Martinez R et al. Stenting for atherosclerotic occlusive disease of the subclavian artery. *Ann Vasc Surg* 1999; **13**:254–60.

9. Whitacker SC, Gregson RH. Case report: occlusion of subclavian artery treated by percutaneous angioplasty. *Clin Radiol* 1991; **44**:199–200.

10. Barbeau GR, Seeger JM, Jablonski S et al. Peripheral artery recanalization in humans using balloon and laser angioplasty. *Clin Cardiol* 1996; **19**:232–8.

11. Schofer J, Rau Th. Schlueter M, Mathey DG. Short-term results and intermediate-term follow-up of laser wire recanalization of chronic coronary artery occlusions: a single center experience. *J Am Coll Cardiol* 1997; **30**:1722–8.

12. Hamburger JN, Gijbers GH, Ozaki Y et al. Recanalization of chronic total coronary occlusions using a laser guide wire: a pilot study. *J Am Coll Cardiol* 1997; **30**:649–56.

13. Sievert H, Rohde S, Eusslen R et al. Recanalization of chronic coronary occlusions using a laser wire. *Cathet Cardiovasc Diagn* 1996; **37**:220–2.

14. Nastur A, Sayers RD, Bell PRF, Bolia A. Protection against vertebral artery embolization during proximal subclavian artery angioplasty. *Eur J Vasc Surg* 1994; **81**:1093–5.

15. Ringelstein EB, Zeumer H. Delayed reversal of vertebral artery blood flow following percutaneous transluminal angioplasty for subclavian steal syndrome. *Neuroradiology* 1984; **26**:189–98.

Case 34

Left Subclavian Artery Stenosis After Left Internal Mammary Artery (LIMA) Bypass Surgery

David R Ramsdale and Serge Osula

Background

A 58-year-old man had severe angina 6 years after coronary artery bypass (CABG) surgery, and noticed that his left hand and arm felt cold. Cardiac catheterization showed a severe stenosis in the left subclavian artery shortly after its origin (Fig. 34.1, arrowhead). The vertebral artery was not visible and the LIMA and rest of the subclavian artery filled only faintly. The stenosis was crossed with a 0.014 inch floppy guidewire and dilated with a 4.0 mm Freeway balloon (JoMed) (Fig. 34.2). This produced significant improvement. The vertebral artery was then visualized and shown to have a severe ostial stenosis (Fig. 34.3, arrowhead) and the LIMA looked normal with fast antegrade flow. The patient noticed immediate warming of the left hand. A 10 × 20 mm long Wallstent (Boston Scientific/Scimed) was then positioned across the stenosis but, on withdrawal of the protective sheath, the shortening self-expanding stent 'melon-seeded' forward so that it only partially covered the stenosis (Fig. 34.4).

An 8 × 30 mm long Powerflex Plus (Cordis/Johnson and Johnson) balloon was then used to further dilate the stent. It was then apparent that the stenosis was very hard and resistant to dilatation (Fig. 34.5) and presumably this had been the reason for the forward displacement of the Wallstent. Local dissection was visible beginning just after the origin of the vertebral artery with associated spasm in the subclavian artery itself (Fig. 34.6). A 17 mm long JoStent Flex (JoMed) stent was then crimped on to a 6 × 20 mm long Bypass Speedy balloon and deployed over the stenosis and overlapping the stents (Fig. 34.7). An 8 × 30 mm long Blue Max balloon was used to postdilate the two stents (Fig. 34.8). This was followed with a 10 × 20 mm long Powerflex Plus balloon at 14 atmospheres (Fig. 34.9). This final result was accepted (Fig. 34.10).

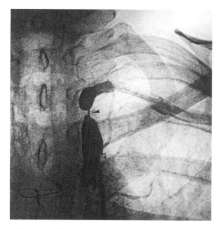

Figure 34.1.

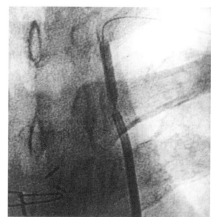

Figure 34.2.

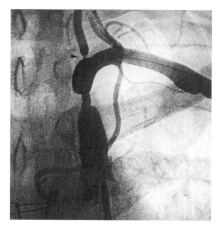

Figure 34.3.

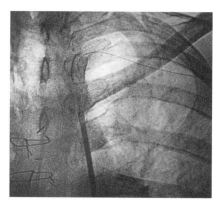

Figure 34.4.

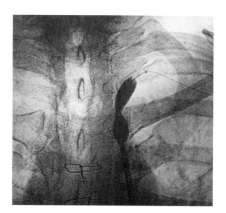

Figure 34.5.

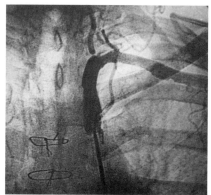

Figure 34.6.

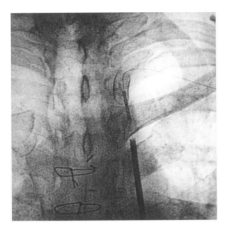

Figure 34.7.

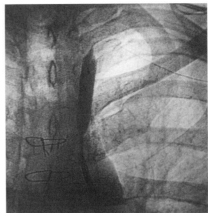

Figure 34.8.

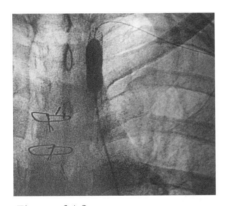

Figure 34.9.

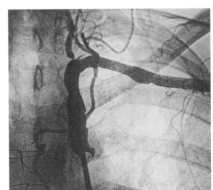

Figure 34.10.

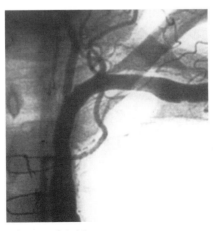

Figure 34.11.

189

The patient's angina improved dramatically and there were no sequelae as a result of the dissection or of the ostial stenosis in the vertebral artery. The decision was made not to stent this non-occlusive tear since this would have resulted in the ostium of the LIMA being covered. At 4 months the dissection was shown to have healed angiographically (Fig. 34.11). The patient remained asymptomatic after 2 years.

Discussion

Atherosclerosis causing critical stenosis in the brachiocephalic or subclavian arteries resulting in the coronary–subclavian steal syndromes (CSSS) is rare, with an estimated incidence of 0.4%.[1] The use of the LIMA in elective bypass grafting of the left anterior descending (LAD) coronary artery is now common practice, but brachiocephalic and subclavian angiography prior to surgical revascularization is not routinely performed. Patients being referred for surgical revascularization of the LAD should be evaluated for cerebrovascular and upper limb ischaemia. The presence of supraclavicular bruits, cold upper-limb extremities, reduced or absent radial pulses and a blood pressure difference >20 mmHg in between the right and left arms should be sought and, if present, subclavian arteriography be performed. Identification of a critical stenosis leaves the surgeon with the options of using the LIMA as a free graft, or using another arterial or venous conduit.[2] There are very few reports in the literature where surgical revascularization or percutaneous transluminal coronary angioplasty (PTCA), with or without the use of stents, has been used to successfully restore myocardial perfusion in patients with CSSS.[3–5] Total occlusions of the left subclavian artery usually requires carotid–subclavian bypass, although a short occlusion might be revascularized by the excimer laser PRIMA wire, PTCA and stent implantation.

Although no series specific for CSSS have been reported, several series of PTCA and stenting for subclavian artery stenosis or occlusion have been published. Henry et al[6] reported a 94% success rate in 135 patients (110 stenosis, 25 occlusions) over a 10-year period. Most patients had upper-limb ischaemia (51.8%), vertebrobasilar insufficiency (53.3%) or both (22.2%), with only nine patients (6.6%) having coronary steal. They had a 1.5% procedural complication rate (one transient ischaemic attack, one fatal stroke and two arterial thromboses) and a 14% restenosis rate. There was little difference in the restenosis rate between the stented and non-stented patients. Although these and other workers have documented only limited success rates for total occlusions, others claim a 94% success rate.[7]

190

Whether self-expanding or balloon-expandable stents are the most appropriate in this situation remains to be determined. The former, such as the Wallstent, have the disadvantage of significant shortening on deployment, and some concern has also been expressed about their use in the more peripheral part of the subclavian artery where they may be prone to flexion and compression forces.[8]

In our case, symptoms of peripheral vascular disease first occurred 8 years after CABG surgery. This suggests progression of atherosclerosis and reinforces the importance of risk-factor modulation where possible. The syndrome of a cold left hand and return of angina following a LIMA graft is specific enough to identify the site of the vascular pathology and requires urgent investigation and treatment.

References

1. Rossum AC, Weinstein E, Holland M. Angiographic evaluation of a carotid–subclavian bypass graft in a patient with subclavian artery stenosis and left internal mammary bypass graft. *Cathet Cardiovasc Diagn* 1994; **32**:178–81.

2. Marshall Jr WG, Miller EC, Kouchoukos NT. The coronary–subclavian steal syndrome: report of a case and recommendations for prevention and management. *Ann Thorac Surg* 1988; **48**:93–6.

3. Kugelmass AD, Kim D, Kuntz RE et al. Endoluminal stenting of a subclavian artery stenosis to treat ischaemia in the distribution of a patent left internal mammary graft. *Cathet Cardiovasc Diagn* 1994; **33**:175–7.

4. Diethrich EB, Cozacov JC. Subclavian stent implantation to alleviate coronary steal through a patent internal mammary graft. *J Endovasc Surg* 1995; **2**:77–80.

5. Sandison AJ, Panayiotopoulos YP, Corr LA et al. Recurrent coronary–subclavian steal syndrome treated by left subclavian artery stenting. *Eur J Endovasc Surg* 1997; **14**:403–5.

6. Henry M, Amor M, Henry I et al. Endoluminal treatment of subclavian occlusive diseases: percutaneous angioplasty and stenting. *Eur Heart J* 1999; **20**(abstract):133(Suppl).

7. Martinez R, Rodriguez-Lopez J, Torruella L et al. Stenting for occlusion of the subclavian arteries. Technical aspects and follow-up results. *Tex Heart Inst J* 1997; **24**:23–7.

8. Phipp LH, Scott DJ, Kessel D et al. Subclavian stents and stent grafts: cause for concern? *J Endovasc Surg* 1999; **6**:223–6.

191

Case 35

INTERMEDIATE LESIONS MAY LOOK THE SAME BUT ASSESSMENT OF FRACTIONAL FLOW RESERVE (FFR) MAY HELP TO DIFFERENTIATE THEM

Bernard de Bruyne and Glenn van Langenhove

Background

RU is a 52-year old engineer. For a few weeks prior to admission, the patient complained of a vague burning sensation during jogging. He was admitted because he sustained an aborted sudden death while watching television a few hours after jogging. Ventricular fibrillation was diagnosed and treated by cardiopulmonary resuscitation and electrical cardioversion.

At admission, the electrocardiogram (ECG) showed non-specific repolarization abnormalities but no obvious signs of ischemia.

The left ventricular (LV) angiogram performed 2 days after the acute episode showed a mild hypokinesia of the anterior wall with an asynchronous relaxation pattern.

The coronary angiogram showed diffuse mild irregularities with a 41% diameter stenosis [minimal luminal diameter (MLD) of 2.3 mm] in the proximal left anterior descending (LAD) artery (Fig. 35.1). When passing a pressure wire through this segment a sudden pressure drop of 35 mmHg was observed (Fig. 35.2a). The latter further increased to 52 mmHg after adenosine administration (18 μg intracoronary), corresponding to an FFR of 0.53 (Fig. 35.2b).

The FFR is calculated as the ratio of the coronary pressure distal to the stenosis over the proximal coronary pressure during maximal hyperemia and decreases as the severity of the stenosis increases. The threshold value for hemodynamic significance is 0.75. Therefore, stent implantation was performed with a good result.

Six months later, the patient had remained asymptomatic and his exercise ECG was normal. At repeat catheterization, the LV angiogram was normal

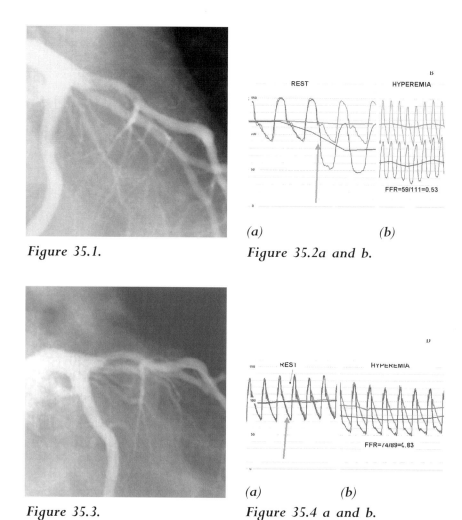

Figure 35.1.

(a) *(b)*

Figure 35.2a and b.

Figure 35.3.

(a) *(b)*

Figure 35.4 a and b.

and the coronary angiogram showed moderate in-stent restenosis (44% diameter stenosis and MLD of 2.3 mm), quite similar to the initial angiographic analysis (Fig. 35.3). Nevertheless, the pressure wire measurement revealed no noticeable gradient at rest and the gradient during hyperemia was 15 mmHg, corresponding to an FFR of 0.83 [Fig. 35.4a shows pressure gradient on crossing lesion (arrow), and (b) shows the hyperemic response.]

This case illustrates the fact that although stenoses may have similar angiographic appearances hemodynamic significances can be strikingly different.

194

Case 36

Physiologic Significance Of The Simultaneous Measurement Of Coronary Flow Reserve (CFR) And Fractional Flow Reserve (FFR) During Complex Stenting Of The Left Anterior Descending (LAD) Artery

Eugenia Nikolsky, Chanderashekhar Patil and Raphael Beyar

Background

A 69-year-old hypertensive male was referred for repeat coronary angiography following unstable angina (Braunwald class IIB2) and thallium perfusion imaging indicating ischemia in the anteroseptal wall. He had a history of diaphragmatic myocardial infarction 8 months previously, treated with primary coronary angioplasty with stent implantation to the proximal portion of the left circumflex (LCx) artery. Repeat balloon angioplasty to the same vessel, due to in-stent restenosis, was performed 4 months after stent implantation, 3 months prior to the current hospitalization. Physical examination on admission was normal. An electrocardiogram (ECG) showed a normal sinus rhythm but signs of left ventricular (LV) hypertrophy. Echocardiography showed a normal global LV systolic function. His medical treatment included daily aspirin, metoprolol and fosinopril.

The diagnostic angiographic study was followed by an assessment of coronary artery lesion severity using the Florence Medical's SmartFlow system.[1,2] This system utilizes computational fluid dynamics to calculate simultaneously both the FFR and the CFR from the pressure signal obtained with a single pressure-monitoring guidewire (RADI Medical Systems, Sweden). The methodology of pressure-based CFR measurements is described elsewhere,[1–3] but, in principle, obtaining proximal and distal coronary pressures at baseline and maximum myocardial hyperemia, and assuming the well-known quadratic relationship between pressure gradient and flow, the CFR is calculated by:

$$CFR = (Qhyper)_{max}/(Qrest)_{max} = \sqrt{(HPG_{max}/BPG_{max})},$$

where BPG and HPG are base and hyperemic pressure gradients, respectively, and $_{max}$ relates to the time of maximal diastolic flow.

Discussion

We present here a case of percutaneous coronary intervention (PCI) where the clinical assessment and then the decision regarding the revascularization procedure were carried out based on a combined anatomical/physiological approach, using the Florence Medical's SmartFlow system to measure both the FFR and the pressure-derived CFR throughout the procedure. Coronary angiography showed severe stenosis in the proximal segment of the LAD and an intermediate lesion in the middle portion of the LAD (Fig. 36.1). After the proximal stenosis was successfully dilated and stented, the FFR improved from 0.42 to 0.67, still reflecting a significant residual hyperemic trans-stenotic gradient (Fig. 36.2). Similarly, the calculated CFR increased from 1.05 to 1.4. Only after the second lesion was dilated and stented (Fig. 36.3) did the FFR

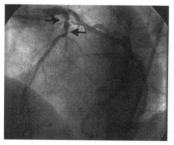
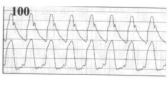

Figure 36.1. *Coronary angiogram shows patent stent in the LCx artery, a 90% stenosis in the proximal portion of the 3.0 mm LAD (upper arrow) and an intermediate lesion (55% diameter stenosis by quantitative coronary angiography, lower arrow) in its middle portion. Right panel: according to the Florence Medical's SmartFlow system, both the FFR and the CFR were severely reduced (0.42 and 1.05, respectively): upper trace, proximal coronary pressure; lower trace, distal coronary pressure; both with adenosine stress.*

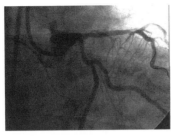
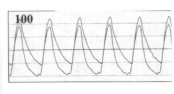

Figure 36.2. *Percutaneous transluminal coronary angioplasty (PTCA) to the proximal lesion in the LAD using a 2.5 mm balloon and subsequent BioDivysio (3 × 15 mm) stent deployment was performed with a good angiographic result. The pressure tracings (right panel) still showed a hyperemic trans-stenotic pressure gradient, with a calculated FFR value of 0.67; the CFR at this stage was 1.4.*

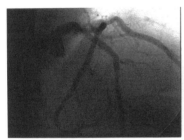
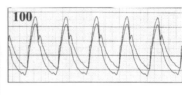

Figure 36.3. *Assuming that the lesion in the middle portion of the LAD was responsible for the remaining gradient, the lesion was dilated and an AVE (3 × 15 mm) stent was implanted. The FFR after the procedure increased to 0.89, but the CFR was still low (1.32).*

increase to a normal value (0.89). Notably, despite an adequate angiographic result, no significant improvement in the CFR was achieved (CFR = 1.32), suggesting an impaired vascular bed response. Six hours after the end of the procedure, severe chest pain and 12-lead ECG changes, compatible with acute myocardial infarction (AMI) in the anterior wall, were followed by an emergency coronary angiography. The latter revealed total occlusion of the LAD following acute thrombosis in the region of the proximal stent (Fig. 36.4). The patient was given IV abciximab and percutaneous balloon dilatation was performed, restoring the blood flow in the LAD (Fig. 36.5).

This case demonstrates that it can be impossible to assess precisely the severity of a lesion from coronary angiography alone. The limitation of coronary angiography is well known: it remains inexact, especially in the estimation of intermediate lesions. Therefore, to assess properly the severity

197

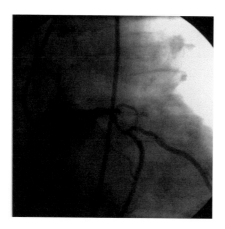

Figure 36.4. *Repeat angiography of the left coronary artery (LCA) 6 hours after the end of the first procedure, due to severe chest pain and ST elevation in the anterior leads of the ECG. Note the total occlusion of the proximal portion of the LAD compatible with acute stent thrombosis.*

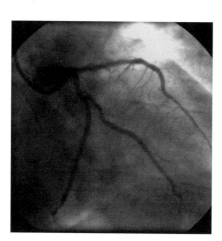

Figure 36.5. *The final result after rescue balloon angioplasty. The patient had a stormy course following the procedure, but eventually stabilized and was discharged home.*

of the stenosis, the angiographic study was complemented with physiological data. An approach that takes into account both anatomic and functional data in clinical decision-making has been investigated in a series of studies, using the measurement of myocardial FFR, demonstrating obvious advantages compared to the anatomic approach only.[4–6] The studies of translesional coronary physiology showed that myocardial FFR has a high correlation with non-invasive techniques assessing ischemia (exercise stress test, thallium scintigraphy and stress dobutamine echocardiography,[7–10] and may reliably predict the clinical outcome in patients with intermediate lesions and identify those patients with a low cardiac event rate.[11–16]

One of the most feasible and safest methods to quickly obtain important coronary physiologic information is the use of myocardial FFR, based on the measurements of translesional pressure gradients by applying a pressure-monitoring intracoronary guidewire. In our case, we used this wire for the pressure signal and based on computational fluid dynamics, the Florence Medical's SmartFlow[1,2] system, calculated the CFR simultaneously. Obtaining both measurements at the same time provides important information regarding the precise functional assessment of the epicardial stenosis (i.e. FFR) and of the distal microcirculation (i.e. CFR).[17] The absence of an improvement in the CFR in this case, despite a good final angiographic result and an obvious increase in the FFR, tends to assume that a significant microvascular disorder possibly played the role in the development of acute stent thrombosis.

In summary, this case emphasizes the value of combining an anatomical and a pressure-based physiological approach in the proper assessment of the significance of the angiographic findings and clinical decision-making before, and throughout, an interventional procedure.

References

1. Gruberg L, Mintz G, Fuchs S et al. Simultaneous assessment of coronary flow reserve and fractional flow reserve with a novel pressure-based method. *J Intervent Cardiol* 2000; **13**:323–30.

2. Shalman E, Barak K, Dgany E et al. Pressure based simultaneous CFR and FFR measurements: understanding the physiology of a stenosed vessel. *Comp Biol Med* 2001; **31**:353–63.

3. Young DF, Tsai FY. Flow characteristics in model of arterial stenosis. II. Unsteady flow. *J Biomech* 1973; **6**:547–59.

4. Pijls NHJ, De Bruyne B, Peels K et al. Measurement of myocardial fractional flow reserve to assess the functional severity of coronary artery stenosis. *N Engl J Med* 1996; **334**:1703–8.

5. Serruys PW, di Mario C, Piek J et al, for the DEBATE study group. Prognostic value of intracoronary low velocity and diameter stenosis in assessing the short- and long-term outcomes of coronary balloon angioplasty: the DEBATE study (Doppler Endpoints Balloon Angioplasty Trial Europe). *Circulation* 1997; **96**:3369–77.

6. Baumgart D, Haude M, Goege G et al. Improved assessment of coronary stenosis severity using the relative flow velocity reserve. *Circulation* 1998; **98**:40–6.

7. Schulman DS, Lasorda D, Farah T et al. Correlations between coronary flow reserve measured with a Doppler guide wire and treadmill exercise testing. *Am Heart J* 1997; **134**:99–104.

8. Donohue TJ, Miller DD, Bach RG et al. Correlation of poststenotic hyperemic coronary flow velocity and pressure with abnormal stress myocardial perfusion imaging in coronary artery disease. *Am J Cardiol* 1997; **77**:948–54.

9. De Bruyne B, Bartunek J, Sys SU, Heyndrickx GR. Relation between myocardial fractional flow reserve calculated from coronary pressure measurements and exercise-induced myocardial ischemia. *Circulation* 1995; **92**:39–46.

10. Bartunek J, Van Schuerbeeck E, De Bruyne B. Comparison of exercise electrocardiography and dobutamine echocardiography with invasively assessed myocardial fractional flow reserve in evaluation of severity of coronary arterial narrowing. *Am J Cardiol* 1997; **79**:478–81.

11. Kern MJ, Donohue TJ, Aguirre FV et al. Clinical outcome of deferring angioplasty in patients with normal translesional pressure-flow velocity measurements. *J Am Coll Cardiol* 1995; **25**: 178–87.

12. Ferrari M, Schnell B, Werner GS, Figulla HR. Safety of deferring angioplasty in patients with normal coronary flow reserve. *J Am Coll Cardiol* 1999; **33**:83–7.

13. Bech GJ, De Bruyne B, Bonnier HJRM et al. Long-term follow-up after deferral of percutaneous transluminal coronary angioplasty of intermediate stenosis on the basis of coronary pressure measurement. *J Am Coll Cardiol* 1998; **31**:841–7.

14. Lesser JL, Wilson RF, White CW. Physiologic assessment of coronary stenoses of intermediate severity can facilitate patient selection for coronary angioplasty. *J Coron Art Dis* 1990; **1**:697–705.

15. Gruberg L, Kapeliovich M, Roguin A et al. Deferring angioplasty in intermediate coronary lesions based on coronary flow criteria is safe: comparison of a deferred group to intervention group. *Int J Cardiovasc Intervent* 1999; **2**:35–40.

16. Bech GJ, NHJ Pijls, Bruyne B et al. Usefulness of fractional flow reserve to predict clinical outcome after balloon angioplasty. *Circulation* 1999; **99**:883–8.

17. Pijls NHJ, Kern MJ, Yock PG, Bruyne B. Practice and potential pitfalls of coronary pressure measurement. *Cathet Cardiovasc Intervent* 2000; **49**:1–16.

Case 37

Intermediate Lesions Analysis In Three-Vessel Disease (3VD) To Allow 2VD Percutaneous Coronary Intervention (PCI)

John McB Hodgson

Background

The patient was a 72-year-old woman with angina pectoris (Canadian class 3) and multiple medical problems. A dobutamine stress echo revealed mid-inferior ischemia and a fixed scar in the basal inferior segment. Her global ejection fraction (EF) was 55%. She was referred for catheterization with possible intervention.

Other medical problems included morbid obesity (125 kg, 152 cm), hypertension, diabetes, gout, osteoarthritis and a distant history of rheumatic heart disease. Surgical history included three abdominal surgeries (appendectomy, hysterectomy, umbilical hernia repair). Her medications were: metoprolol, omperazole, glyburide, diuretics, lisinopril, allopurinol, colchicine, isosorbide mononitrate, celecoxib and aspirin.

Cardiac catheterization commentary

Right and left heart cardiac catheterization was performed using the Judkins technique. The left ventricular end diastolic pressure was 20 mmHg. Right heart pressures were moderately elevated (pulmonary artery 44/24 mmHg, right atrium 12 mmHg mean). Pulmonary vascular resistance was elevated at 3.2 Wood units. Simultaneous measurement showed no aortic or mitral valve gradients. Oxygen saturations showed no intracardiac shunt. Biplane left venticulography demonstrated inferobasal and posterolateral akinesis with a global EF of 70%.

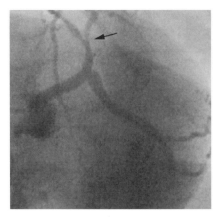

Figure 37.1. *Left anterior oblique (LAO) caudal projection of the left coronary artery (LCA) showing the LAD/diagonal lesion.*

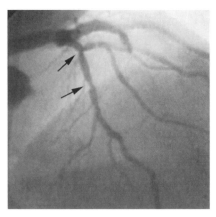

Figure 37.2. *AP cranial projection of the LCA showing the additional mid-LAD lesion.*

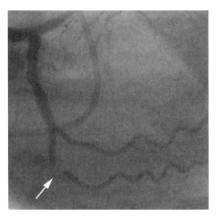

Figure 37.3. *Right anterior oblique (RAO) caudal projection showing the LCx lesion.*

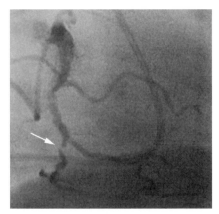

Figure 37.4. *RAO projection of the RCA showing the distal lesion.*

Coronary angiography revealed coronary calcification. The left main was not significantly involved. The left anterior descending (LAD) artery had diffuse disease in the proximal portion, involving a large diagonal branch (Figs 37.1 and 37.2). The mid-LAD had a 60% focal lesion (Fig. 37.2). The left circumflex (LCx) had a focal subtotal ostial lesion of the third obtuse marginal (OM3) (Fig. 37.3). The right coronary artery (RCA) was dominant and had diffuse mid-vessel disease with a 90% focal lesion in the distal third (Fig. 37.4).

Discussion

This patient presents a common therapeutic dilemma: an elderly, obese, diabetic woman with 3VD. The proper management of such patients is still unclear. While some studies (most notably BARI) have suggested improved long-term outcome with coronary artery bypass graft (CABG) surgery rather than PCI, many interventionalists believe that multivessel-PCI is a reasonable alternative. It was our impression that this particular patient presented a high risk for surgery and was likely to have a protracted postoperative recovery period. We therefore utilized additional catheter-based techniques to assist in the triage decision.

Since the LAD disease appeared to be the least severe, we utilized translesional pressure measurements to assess the physiologic significance of these lesions. Our intention was to proceed with surgery if the LAD disease was significant and to perform two-vessel PCI if it was not. The fractional flow reserve (FFR) was determined using a JOMED Wavewire, and intracoronary adenosine boluses (24–48 µg): the FFR in the LAD, distal to all lesions, was 0.85 (Fig. 37.7) and in the diagonal was 0.87 (Fig. 37.8). Both values are well above the 0.75 threshold for ischemia. Several studies have shown that when the FFR is >0.75 then deferral of intervention is safe and associated with a low incidence of recurrent events (<10%).

Based on the FFR results, PCI was undertaken at the same setting. The Cx lesion was primarily stented (2.75 × 8 mm; Fig. 37.5) and the RCA was treated with a cutting balloon (2.5 × 10 mm; Fig. 37.6). The patient was discharged the following morning without complication.

At 5 months follow-up the patient remained free of angina: her cholesterol was 157 mg/dl with a high-density lipoprotein (HDL) fraction of 52 mg/dl.

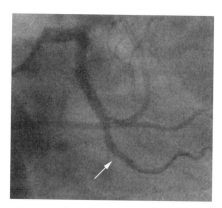

Figure 37.5. Cx following stent placement.

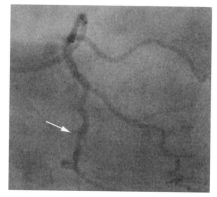

Figure 37.6. RCA following cutting balloon.

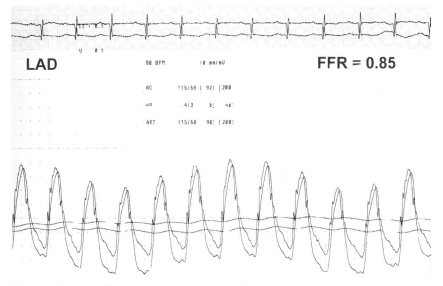

Figure 37.7. *FFR determination in the LAD.*

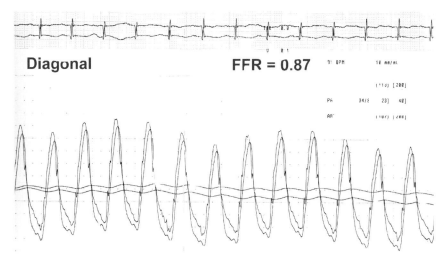

Figure 37.8. *FFR determination in the diagonal.*

Further reading

Niles NW, McGrath PD, Malenka D et al. Survival of patients with diabetes and multivessel coronary artery disease after surgical or percutaneous coronary revascularization: results of a large regional prospective study. *J Am Coll Cardiol* 2001; **37**:1008–15.

Best PJM, Berger PB. Has the surgical era ended for multivessel coronary artery disease? A treatment update. *Appl Imaging* 2001; **Nov**: 5–12.

Pijls NHJ, Van Gelder B, Van der Voort P et al. Fractional Flow Reserve: a useful index to evaluate the influence of an epicardial coronary stenosis on myocardial blood flow. *Circulation* 1995; **92**:3183–93.

Pijls NHJ, de Bruyne B, Peels et al. Measurement of myocardial fractional flow reserve to assess the functional severity of coronary artery stenosis. *N Engl J Med* 1996; **34**:1703–8.

Bech GJW, de Bruyne B, Bartunek J et al. Long term follow-up after deferral of percutaneous transluminal coronary angioplasty of intermediate stenoses on the basis of coronary pressure measurement. *J Am Coll Cardiol* 1998; **31**:841–7.

Bech GJW, deBruyne B, Pijls NHJ et al. Fractional flow reserve to determine the appropriateness of angioplasty in moderate coronary stenosis. A randomized trial. *Circulation* 2001; **103**:2928–34.

Bech GJW, Droste H, Pijls NHJ et al. Value of fractional flow reserve in making decisions about bypass surgery for equivocal left main coronary artery disease. *Heart* 2001; **86**:547–52.

Case 38

IMPLANTATION OF A NEW SIROLIMUS-COATED STENT GUIDED BY INTRAVASCULAR ULTRASOUND (IVUS): A POTENTIAL CURE OF RESTENOSIS

Marco A Costa, Alexandre Abizaid, Andrea S Abizaid,
R Staico, A Chaves, M Centemero, ACS Silva,
Amanda GMR Sousa and J Eduardo Sousa

Clinical history

A 47-year-old male was referred to our institution after an episode of angina at rest. He had had an anterior myocardial infarction treated with streptokinase 20 days prior to admission. His risk factors included current smoking and hypercholesterolemia. Angiography showed a moderate (65% diameter stenosis) eccentric stenosis in the mid-left anterior descending (LAD) artery (Fig. 38.1a). The left circumflex (LCx) and right coronary arteries (RCA) were free of significant disease. The reference vessel diameter by QCA was 3.2 mm. Before intervention, IVUS imaging was performed, which revealed an eccentric soft plaque with a lipid core and a minimum lumen (cross-sectional) area (MLA) of 3.0 mm² (Fig. 38.1b). Positive vascular remodeling at the lesion site was also noted. Stent implantation was indicated based on clinical grounds, and IVUS-proven lesion severity and instability. After predilatation using a 3.0 × 16 mm angioplasty balloon, a 3.5 × 18 mm sirolimus-coated Bx Velocity stent was deployed at 16 atmospheres. No postdilatation was required, since post-stenting IVUS interrogation showed good stent apposition with an MLA >90% of the mean reference lumen cross-sectional area. The patient was discharged the following day, on clopidogrel 75 mg a day for 60 days. After 4 months he was free of angina and returned for a control angiographic and IVUS follow-up. There was no lumen loss observed by angiography, whereas IVUS revealed a complete absence of neointimal hyperplasia throughout the stent (Fig. 38.2).

207

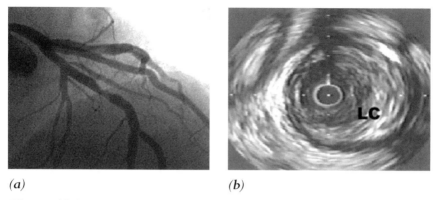

(a)   *(b)*

Figure 38.1. *Pre-procedure angiography (a) and IVUS (b) imaging. Angiography shows a moderate lesion in the mid-portion of the LAD. IVUS revealed a soft, eccentric plaque with a lipid core (LC). The elliptic shape of the external elastic membrane (EEM), specifically at the side of lesion, may suggest adaptive vascular remodeling, which was confirmed by quantitative measurements (EEM area at the lesion site > mean reference EEM area).*

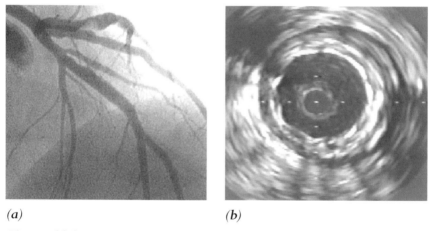

(a)   *(b)*

Figure 38.2. *Follow-up angiography (a) and IVUS (b) imaging.*

Comments

This case illustrates the value of IVUS imaging in determining lesion severity and plaque instability. Based on angiography, one may question the physiological significance of this moderate mid-LAD lesion. Previous reports have described a close relationship between IVUS anatomical parameters and

208

the hemodynamic significance of a given coronary stenosis.[1–3] Recently, IVUS studies have demonstrated that a lesion with an MLA $>4.0 \, mm^2$ was associated with a coronary flow reserve (CFR) >2.0.[1,2] Thus, the $3.0 \, mm^2$ MLA suggested the physiological importance of this moderate lesion. Furthermore, IVUS detection of a lipid core and positive remodeling may suggest plaque instability, as reported previously. The concept of sealing unstable plaques by stent implantation may also be a plausible indication for intervention in this case, although this hypothesis needs to be established by clinical studies.

The second major observation that arises from this case is the complete absence of neointimal proliferation at follow-up. The use of a sirolimus-coated stent in this patient may have contributed to this finding. Sirolimus (rapamycin; Rapamune), a natural macrocyclic lactone, is a potent immunosuppressive agent that was developed by Wyeth-Ayerst Laboratories and approved by the Food and Drug Administration (FDA) for the prophylaxis of renal transplant rejection in 1999. This drug induces cell-cycle arrest in the late G1 phase. It inhibits proliferation of both rat and human smooth muscle cells in vitro[4,5] and reduces intimal thickening in models of vascular injury.[6,7] Polymer coating allows controlled release of the medication at the site of vascular injury for a period >15 days. Combined with the scaffold properties of tubular stents, this new antiproliferative drug-coated stent has the potential of blocking the two major components of the restenotic process, i.e. intimal hyperplasia and negative remodeling.

This patient was enrolled in the first series of patients treated with the sirolimus-coated Bx Velocity stent worldwide. The safety and feasibility of the implantation of this new stent has recently been demonstrated. In this pioneer investigation, including 30 patients, only a minimal amount of neointimal proliferation was detected by IVUS.[8] If these results are confirmed in randomized trials, this new generation of coronary stents will become a breakthrough in interventional cardiology.

References

1. Abizaid A, Mintz GS, Pichard AD et al. Clinical, intravascular ultrasound, and quantitative angiographic determinants of the coronary flow reserve before and after percutaneous transluminal coronary angioplasty. Am J Cardiol 1998; 82:423–8.

2. Abizaid AS, Mintz GS, Mehran R et al. Long-term follow-up after percutaneous transluminal coronary angioplasty was not performed based on intravascular ultrasound findings: importance of lumen dimensions. Circulation 1999; 100:256–61.

209

3. Takagi A, Tsurumi Y, Ishii Y et al. Clinical potential of intravascular ultrasound for physiological assessment of coronary stenosis: relationship between quantitative ultrasound tomography and pressure-derived fractional flow reserve. *Circulation* 1999;**100**:250–5.

4. Poon M, Marx SO, Gallo R et al. Rapamycin inhibits vascular smooth muscle cell migration. *J Clin Invest* 1996; **98**:2277–83.

5. Marx SO, Jayaraman T, Go LO, Marks AR. Rapamycin-FKBP inhibits cell cycle regulators of proliferation in vascular smooth muscle cells. *Circ Res* 1995; **76**:412–17.

6. Gregory CR, Huang X, Pratt RE et al. Treatment with rapamycin and mycophenolic acid reduces arterial intimal thickening produced by mechanical injury and allows endothelial replacement. *Transplantation* 1995; **59**:655–61.

7. Gallo R, Padurean A, Jayaraman T et al. Inhibition of intimal thickening after balloon angioplasty in porcine coronary arteries by targeting regulators of the cell cycle. *Circulation* 1999; **99**:2164–70.

8. Sousa JMR, Abizaid AAC, Abizaid ACLS et al. First human experience with sirolimus-coated Bx velocity stent: clinical, angiographic and ultrasound late results. *Circulation* 2000; **102**:II–815 (abstract).

Case 39

A CASE OF DRUG-ELUTING STENT DEPLOYMENT

Anthony H Gershlick

Clinical background

The images shown for this case are of a 52-year-old male who presented with stable symptoms of angina. He underwent exercise stress testing, which was positive, and angiography because of on-going symptoms, despite medical therapy with a beta-blocker (atenolol 100 mg od) and isosorbide mononitrate (Imdur 30 mg bid). He had smoked cigars (> five per day) for many years but had stopped 2 years earlier. A recent total cholesterol measurement was 4.7 mmol/l.

Angiographic images

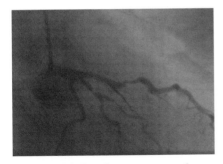 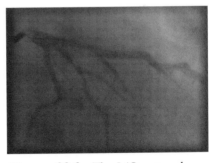

Figure 39.1. The angiogram shows two lesions, one in the left anterior descending (LAD) artery and a tight discrete lesion in the intermediate vessel.

Figure 39.2. The LAD artery has been stented with a **Taxol-eluting stent** as part of the ELUTES (EvaLUation of Taxol-Eluting Stent) trial. The intermediate vessel was stented at the same sitting with a Tetra 3.00 × 13 mm normal, non-eluting stent.

211

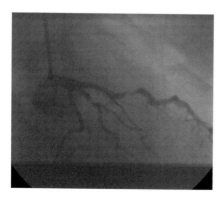

Figure 39.3. Follow-up angiogram at 6 months. This patient was the first to receive a Taxol-eluting stent and is included in the ELUTES trial.

Commentary

Angiographic recurrence after plain old balloon angioplasty (POBA) is noted in up to 35% of patients. The restenotic process is composed of a combination of recoil, negative remodelling and intimal smooth muscle cell hyperplasia. Two benchmark trials, the BENESTENT and STRESS studies, showed that deployment of a stent reduces the chances of restenosis to between 10 and 15%. Stents do this by reducing the impact of recoil and negative remodelling, and by creating a larger initial lumen, allowing more room for the intimal hyperplasia to form. However, stents do not prevent the formation of intimal hyperplasia. When stents restenose, treatment is difficult. Reballooning is quick and easy but leads to re-restenosis in up to 60% of those treated, mostly because achieving a small residual stenosis after balloon angioplasty in the presence of only partially compressible smooth muscle cells is difficult. Atherectomy, at one time thought to be the answer, has not been shown to be any better than balloon angioplasty alone in the ARTIST trial. Vascular brachytherapy has been shown to prevent re-recurrence, but is not without its problems, including geographical miss, edge effects and potential stent thrombosis. Additionally, vascular brachytherapy is a secondary prevention, meaning that the patient has to undergo stent implantation first and the secondary treatment thereafter.

Discussion

There is much current interest in primary prevention of intimal hyperplasia by using the stent as a platform to deliver drugs. There are a number of ongoing clinical trials of drug-based stent delivery. Rapamycin, an agent used in renal transplantation, is being tested on the Cordis Bx Velocity stent, batimistat on the BioDyvisio stent (Biocompatibles plc) and paclitaxol, a chemotherapeutic agent, is being trialled on both the Quantum stent (the SCORES trial) and, as in this case, on the Cook V-flex stent as part of the ELUTES trial. In this trial, four doses of paclitaxol are being compared with control. A total of 180 patients are being randomized to determine the most appropriate dose. The endpoints are angiographic diameter stenosis and major adverse coronary events (MACE) at 6 months. A pivotal trial will be started if needed once the difference between groups has been demonstrated. Long-term follow-up and angiography at 2 years is planned. Should these agents prove to be effective and, most importantly, safe then the era of stent-based drug delivery will have commenced and will be the next quantum leap in percutaneous intervention.

Case 40

THE SHORT-LIVED PROMISE OF THE RADIOACTIVE STENT

Wim J van der Giessen, Evelyn Regar, Jurgen M Ligthart and Patrick W Serruys

Background

The radioactive stent has been put forward as an easy-to-use equivalent of stent implantation followed by catheter-based brachytherapy.[1-3] This proved not to be true. Although the radioactive stent proved very effective in reducing in-stent tissue growth, significant stenosis at the edges limits their widespread use.[4] This case attempts to illustrate this. Furthermore, it shows an intravascular ultrasound (IVUS) appearance so far not seen outside the use of endovascular radiation.

Case description

A 53-year-old male was admitted to hospital with an acute non-Q-wave inferior infarction [maximum creatine kinase (CK) 554 IU/l, $n < 100$ IU/l]. An electrocardiogram (ECG) showed the sinus rhythm, with right bundle branch block (RBBB); the acute phase was uneventful. During mobilization episodes of chest pain accompanied with $\pm$ 1mm ST depression in leads V4–6 and ST elevation in lead III occurred.

On day 6, coronary angiography revealed a significant stenosis in the right coronary artery (RCA) and an occluded left anterior descending (LAD) with akinesia in the anterior wall of the left ventricle. Hypokinesia was shown inferobasally.

It was decided to perform a percutaneous transluminal coronary angioplasty (PTCA) of the RCA. Viability tests of the anterior wall were proposed to identify the need to perform a recanalization of the LAD later.

The patient consented to be enrolled in a phase 1 trial investigating P-32 radioactive stents. This stent (4.0 × 23 mm) was implanted successfully after

215

predilation with a 3.0 × 20 mm balloon under IVUS guidance (Figs 40.1a and b). Anginal episodes became virtually absent after this procedure. After discharge, viability was proven in the anterior wall using dobutamine stress testing. Five weeks after implantation of the radioactive stent the LAD was recanalized successfully and a non-radioactive stent implanted. During the second procedure selective contrast injections in the RCA showed a patent P-32 stent with minimal tissue response (Fig. 40.1c).

Three months after the first procedure the patient started to experience recurrence of angina. An exercise test was positive. At 18 weeks after the

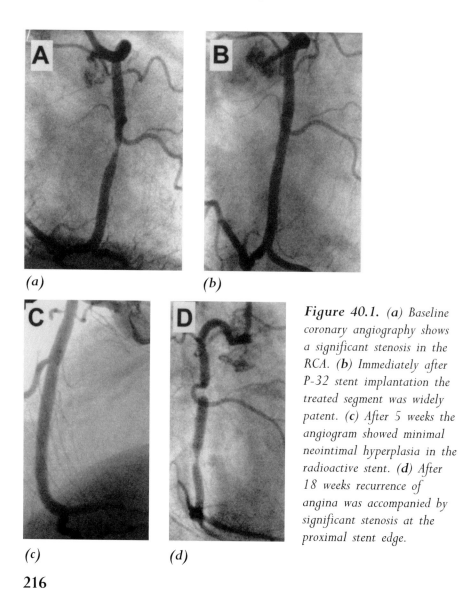

Figure 40.1. (*a*) *Baseline coronary angiography shows a significant stenosis in the RCA.* (*b*) *Immediately after P-32 stent implantation the treated segment was widely patent.* (*c*) *After 5 weeks the angiogram showed minimal neointimal hyperplasia in the radioactive stent.* (*d*) *After 18 weeks recurrence of angina was accompanied by significant stenosis at the proximal stent edge.*

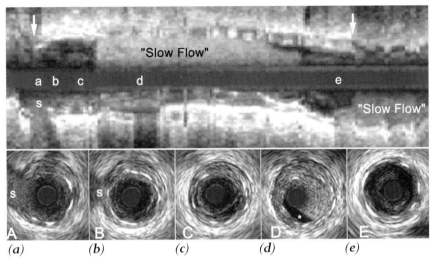

Figure 40.2. *IVUS acquisition at 18 weeks post stent-implantation. The top panel shows the longitudinal IVUS reconstruction. 'S' indicates the right ventricular (RV) branch which is bordering the proximal stent edge. The position of the cross-sections are indicated by their corresponding letters. Both edges of the stent are indicated by arrowheads. Cross-sectional panel A shows the proximal edge of the stent near the RV branch (s). Panel B and C: Concentric 'black hole' with fibrous components. The IVUS catheter is blocking the remaining lumen, thereby slowing down the blood flow and trapping the contrast medium more distally, which is visible at panel D (*). Note also the region of slow blood flow visible at the longitudinal reconstruction. Panel E: Concentric 'black hole' at the distal edge of the stent. Note the blood speckling in the lumen.*

radioactive stent implantation a repeat angiography was performed. The radioactive stent in the RCA showed a significant restenosis (candy-wrapper phenomenon; Fig. 40.1d). This was successfully treated with two short stents proximal and distal to the P-32 stent.

Comments

This case illustrates current interventional cardiology practice to treat multivessel, complex coronary disease. In addition, it demonstrates the short-lived efficacy of radioactive stents.[4]

In this case, neointimal hyperplasia was virtually absent in the P-32 stent after 5 weeks but significant (edge) restenosis occurred between 5 and 18 weeks. The mechanism of this edge restenosis is incompletely understood, but recent data indicate that it is caused by a combination of continued presence of the stent and radioactive dose fall-off.[5] The observation of the 'black hole' is unique for endovascular brachytherapy.[6] Comparing the angiographic picture of Fig. 40.1d with the IVUS images of Figs 40.2b, c and e, it is clear that what is black on the IVUS is stenosing the lumen. In our experience, neointimal hyperplasia after percutaneous coronary intervention (PCI) has always been more echogenic. Very proteoglycan-rich neointima, organized thrombus and stagnant contrast medium may all show this echo transparency.

References

1.   Condado J, Waksman R, Gurdiel O et al. Long-term angiographic and clinical outcome after percutaneous transluminal coronary angioplasty and intracoronary radiation therapy in humans. *Circulation* 1997; **96**:727–32.

2.   Teirstein P, Massullo V, Jani S et al. Catheter-based radiotherapy to inhibit restenosis after coronary stenting. *N Engl J Med* 1997; **336**:1697–703.

3.   Wardeh AJ, Kay IP, Sabate M et al. β-Particle-emitting radioactive stent implantation. A safety and feasibility study. *Circulation* 1999; **100**:1684–9.

4.   Albiero R, Nishida T, Adamian M et al. Edge restenosis after implantation of high activity (32)P radioactive beta-emitting stents. *Circulation* 2000; **101**:2454–7.

5.   van der Giessen WJ, Regar E, Harteveld MS et al. The 'Edge effect' of ^{32}p radioactive stents is caused by the combination of (chronic) stent injury and radioactive dose fall-off. *Circulation* 2001; **104**:2236–41.

6.   Kay IP, Lighart JM, Virmani R et al. The black hole: a new IVUS observation after intracoronary radiation. *Circulation* 2000; **102(Suppl II)**:II-568.

Case 41

Treatment Of In-Stent Restenosis Occurring After Stent Implantation And Brachytherapy For Total Occlusion

Pim J de Feijter, Jurgen Ligthart and Benno Rensing

Background

A 58-year-old male was referred because he was experiencing post-myocardial infarction angina pectoris. Six months earlier he sustained a non-Q-wave inferior myocardial infarction with a maximal creatine kinase (CK) release of 800 IU. He was readmitted with chest pain at rest, adequately responding to medical treatment with aspirin, heparin and nitroglycerin, which were administered in addition to previous treatment with a beta-blocker (Selokeen 50 mg daily) and a calcium antagonist (Norvasc 50 mg daily). His electrocardiogram (ECG) did not reveal signs of ischaemia and troponin T was negative. Physical examination was normal and his blood pressure was 120/70 mmHg. An earlier blood test had demonstrated hypercholesterolaemia (8.0 mmol/l), for which he was treated with simvastatin 40 mg daily.

An exercise stress test provoked chest pain and demonstrated ischaemic ST-segment depressions in leads V4–V6 of maximally 2 mm. He was referred for diagnostic angiography which revealed that the proximal segment of the right coronary artery (RCA) was diffusely diseased and that there was a total occlusion at the mid-segment (Fig. 41.1). There appeared to be a small channel after the total occlusion, which facilitated the attempt to cross the total occlusion. The left coronary artery (LCA) demonstrated several non-significant (<50% lumen diameter) obstructions of the left main and left anterior descending (LAD) arteries and side branches of the circumflex (Cx) artery (Figs 41.2–41.4). A rather large septal branch had severe ostial stenosis. The distal vessel segment of the RCA, the posterolateral branch and the right posterior descending (RPD) artery, were filled by collaterals from,

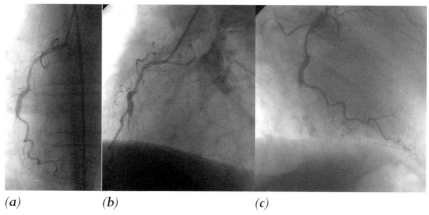

(a)   *(b)*   *(c)*

Figure 41.1. *The RCA is diffusely diseased in its proximal segment (and there is a total occlusion of the mid-segment, which ends in a small 'mouse tail'.* **(a)** *Left anterior oblique (LAO) projection, 10°;* **(b)** *LAO projection, 50°;* **(c)** *right anterior oblique (RAO) projection, 40°.*

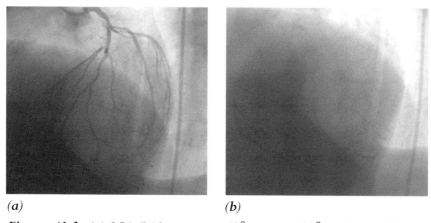

(a)   *(b)*

Figure 41.2. *(a) LCA (LAO projection 40°, superior 30°) with several non-significant stenoses (<50% luminal diameter) in left main LAD and Cx arteries. (b) The large septal branch shows a severe ostial lesion. The distal vessel segments of the RCA are filled by collaterals.*

predominantly, the LAD artery and, to a lesser extent, from the Cx artery. These well-developed vessels were visible up to the crux of the RCA. Hence, the missing occluded vessel segment ran from the mid-segment of the RCA to the crux and was estimated to have a length of several centimetres. The left ventriculogram revealed slight hypokinesia of the inferior wall segments (Fig. 41.5).

220

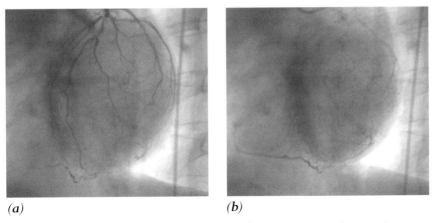

(a)   (b)

Figure 41.3. (a) LCA (LAO projection, 40°) (b) Collateral filling of the distal RCA.

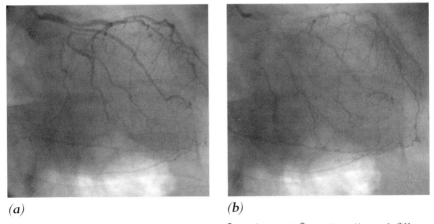

(a)   (b)

Figure 41.4. LCA (RAO projection, 20°, inferior 25°) with collateral filling of the posterolateral branch of the RCA (a) and RPD artery (b); both are visualized until the crux of the RCA.

Percutaneous coronary intervention (PCI) was performed using the bifemoral approach, which allowed simultaneous visualization of the proximal RCA vessel segment before the occlusion and the distal segments after the occlusion (Fig. 41.6). Manipulation of the guiding catheter (Wiseguide JR4) to achieve more catheter support resulted in a proximal occluding dissection of the RCA (Fig. 41.7). The estimated length and course of the missing occluded RCA segment is depicted in Fig. 41.8. Initially, the dissection in the proximal part of the RCA was fixed by a stent implantation (Bx Velocity, 3.5 × 33 mm (Fig. 41.9). It was then relatively easy to cross the

221

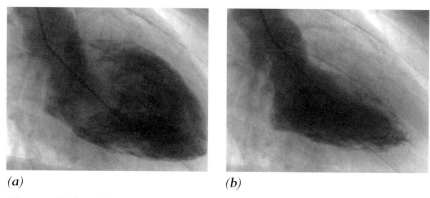

(a)   *(b)*

Figure 41.5. *Left ventriculogram in diastole* **(a)** *and systole* **(b)**. *There is slight hypokinesia of the inferior wall segments.*

Figure 41.6. *Bifemoral simultaneous injection of RCA and LCA (LAO projection, 10°). Proximal diffuse sclerosis and mid-segment RCA with total occlusion. Distal RCA segment filled with collaterals from the LCA. The missing occluded RCA is shown as a white line and is c. 2 cm long.*

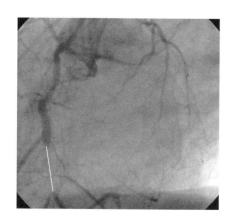

Figure 41.7. *Simultaneous injection in RCA and LCA (LAO projection, 90°).* **(a)** *Proximal and mid-segment RCA is visible with deep seating of the guiding catheter in the RCA.*

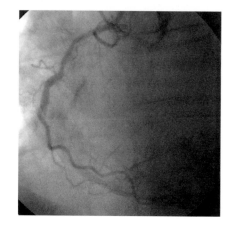

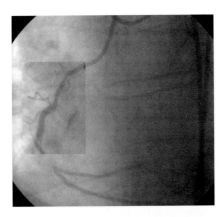

Figure 41.8. Post-processing of Fig. 41.7 allows estimation of the length and course of the 'missing occluded' RCA segment.

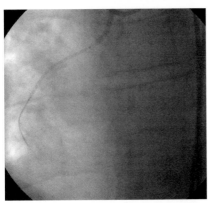

Figure 41.9. Stent implantation (Bx Velocity, 3.5 × 33 mm) of the proximal segment of the diseased and dissected RCA.

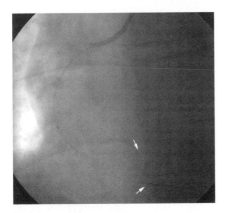

Figure 41.10. Two wires are placed: one in the distal RCA and the other in the acute marginal branch (arrows). The marker of the non-inflated balloon which has crossed the totally occluded segment is clearly visible in the mid-segment of the RCA.

total occlusion and to gain access into the distal vessel lumen using the newest generation guidewires (Terumo Crosswire NT, 0.014 inch, 180 cm). One wire was placed in the distal RCA and another wire in a well-developed acute marginal branch (Fig. 41.10).

223

A non-inflated balloon (Terumo Hayate 2.0 × 20 mm) was passed over the total occluded segment (Fig. 41.10) and withdrawn, demonstrating that antegrade flow was possible and confirming the correct wire location in the distal vessel segment. Thereafter, balloon angioplasty and stent implantation (Bx Velocity, 3.0 × 33 mm) was successfully performed (Fig. 41.11). As part of an ongoing study, brachytherapy was performed using the Novoste Beta Cath 60 mm (Sr90/Y90) (Fig. 41.12). Long-term treatment (1 year) with a combination of aspirin and clopidogrel was given.

However, the patient developed progressive angina after a symptom-free period of c. 4 months. A repeat angiogram demonstrated a totally occluded proximal RCA (Fig. 41.13). The patient was scheduled for another attempt to open the RCA. It was surprisingly easy to cross with the guidewire (PT Graphix Intermediate, 0.014 inch) (Fig. 41.14a), which was facilitated by the presence of the earlier implanted visible stent struts. A non-inflated balloon (Hayate, 1.5 × 20 mm) was passed across the entire occluded segment and withdrawn. A repeat angiogram showed faint antegrade flow and confirmation of the location of the guidewire in the distal vessel segment (Fig. 41.14b). After several inflations of different-sized balloons (Worldpass, 2.0 × 20 mm and 3.0 × 20 mm) the angiographic result was not adequate (Fig. 41.15) and it was decided to re-stent (two Bx Velocity, 3.5 × 33 m, and proximal Bx Velocity, 4.0 × 13 mm) the entire segment, which ended in a satisfactory result (Fig. 41.16). The patient was discharged with continuing clopidogrel medication. The patient was still symptom-free 3 months later.

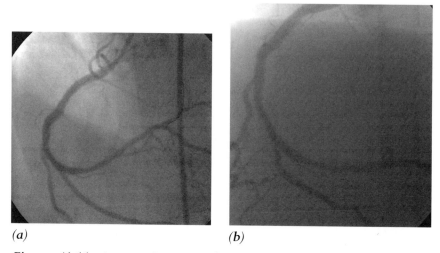

(a) (b)

Figure 41.11. Angiographic result after implantation of two stents (Bx Velocity, 3.5 × 33 mm proximal and Bx Velocity, 3.0 × 33 mm mid-segment RCA): (**a**) LAO projection, superior 15°; (**b**) LAO projection, 25°.

224

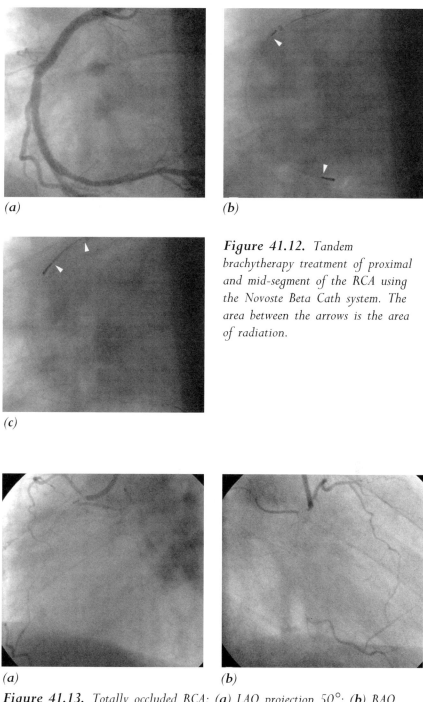

(a)   *(b)*

(c)

Figure 41.12. *Tandem brachytherapy treatment of proximal and mid-segment of the RCA using the Novoste Beta Cath system. The area between the arrows is the area of radiation.*

(a)   *(b)*

Figure 41.13. *Totally occluded RCA: (a) LAO projection 50°; (b) RAO projection, 35°.*

225

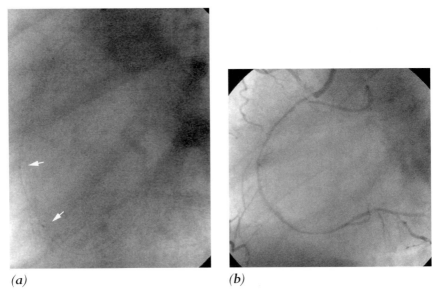

(a)   *(b)*

Figure 41.14. *(a) Wire positioned across the total occlusion in the distal RCA. The contours of the stent struts are faintly visible in the proximal and mid-segment of the RCA. The non-inflated balloon is visible in the mid-segment of the RCA (arrows). (b) Angiogram after having crossed the totally occluded vessel with a non-inflated balloon.*

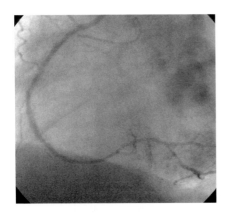

Figure 41.15. *RCA after several inflations with different-sized balloons. The angiographic result is not optimal.*

Discussion

This case history has several interesting aspects. Firstly, how to treat a chronic total occlusion and how to keep this vessel open. Secondly, how to treat diffuse in-stent restenosis, particularly when this occurs after earlier

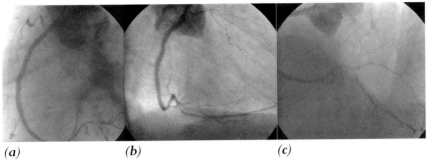

(a)   *(b)*   *(c)*

Figure 41.16. *RCA after repeat implantation of three stents (very proximal Bx Velocity, 4.0 × 13 mm, and proximal and mid: two Bx Velocity, 3.5 × 33 mm). (a) LAO projection, 40°; (b) RAO projection 30°; (c) peripheral segments of the RCA: LAO projection, 40°, superior 30°).*

treatment with brachytherapy. Our approach to treat a chronic total occlusion is clearly demonstrated in this case. It is important to make sure that one obtains a fair idea about the size and length of the distal vessel segment of the occluded vessel, and, importantly, an idea about the length of the 'missing' segment. We prefer a bifemoral approach, whereby both vessels are injected simultaneously. This allows a clear impression of the missing segment and, most importantly, provides a reassuring method to demonstrate that the crossed guidewire is actually within the vessel lumen. It is often difficult, if not impossible, to tell where the guidewire is located, since after an exit (very easily occurring using new guidewires) the guidewire tends to follow the course of the vessel.

Currently, with the availability of very sophisticated guidewire technology, almost all total occlusions may be attempted, the exception being if the distal vessel segment is not visualized (due to diffuse disease) and revascularization is not indicated in the absence of ischaemia and akinesia of segmental left ventricular (LV) contraction. After crossing with the wire we prefer to cross and withdraw a non-deflated small balloon and see whether an injection in the 'occluded' vessel now shows antegrade flow, which 'reconfirms' that the wire is actually within the lumen. This procedure is repeated after inflation at the site of the occlusion. According to the literature, it is now our policy to always perform a stent implantation of a chronically occluded vessel to reduce the likelihood of in-stent restenosis.[1–4] But in this particular case – as part of an ongoing trial investigating the efficacy of additional brachytherapy to further reduce the *c.* 30% occurrence of in-stent restenosis – after stent implantation for chronic total occlusion, brachytherapy was also performed using beta-radiation. This approach may

227

raise an important issue: if upfront brachytherapy fails then one has precluded the only efficacious option to treat in-stent restenosis (i.e. brachytherapy) should restenosis occur, because it is recommended to use brachytherapy only once due to the potential occurrence of late adverse events (late-occurring cell proliferation).[5] These patients should be protected with long-term clopidogrel treatment to prevent late thrombotic occlusion.[6]

Unfortunately, diffuse in-stent restenosis with total occlusion occurred in this patient. This clearly places the treating physician in a dilemma. How to manage this awkward clinical situation? Intensification of medical treatment is the first option, but after consultation with the patient this was not pursued. Bypass surgery with one graft on the RCA is certainly a reasonable consideration, but in this case should be regarded as a last resort. Therefore, we were left with the third option, an attempt to open the totally occluded stented portion of the RCA with the knowledge of a high likelihood of the recurrence of re-re-occlusion.

In in-stent restenosis it is often quite easy to cross with a guidewire because the neointimal tissue is soft and the passage of the wire is facilitated by the visible contours of the stent struts. We considered balloon dilatation as the 'best' option in this situation, since other techniques have not shown superior results in the percutaneous treatment of diffuse in-stent restenosis or re-occlusion. However, as was expected, this resulted in a non-optimal

Table 41.1. Elective stenting versus balloon angioplasty to reduce restenosis

		Chronic total occlusions					
		Restenosis (%)		TVR* (%)		Composite endpoint[†] (%)	
	NP	Stent	Balloon	Stent	Balloon	Stent	Balloon
Trial							
SICCO	117	32	72	21	39	21	46
GISSOC	110	32	68	5	22	n.a.	n.a.
SPACTO	85	33	64	28	45	30	42
TOSCA	410	55	70	9	16	24	24

*Target vessel revascularization.
[†]Composite endpoint: death, myocardial infarction and repeat revascularization; n.a., not available.
SICCO, Stenting in Chronic Coronary Occlusion; GISSOC, Gruppo Italiano di Studio sullo Stent nelle Occlusioni Coronoriche; SPACTO, STent versus PTCA after recanalization of Chronic Total Occlusions; TOSCA, Total Occlusion Study of Canada.

angiographic luminal result and, therefore, the whole trajectory of the proximal and mid-segment of the RCA was again completely stented. The end result was angiographically reasonable, but the likelihood of sustained success is rather low.

After a 3 month follow-up the patient was still symptom-free. Should re-re-re-occlusion occur, and since continued medication is not an option, we will refer the patient, reluctantly, to bypass surgery.

References

1. Buller CE, Dzavik V, Carere RG et al. Primary stenting versus balloon angioplasty in occluded coronary arteries: the Total Occlusion Study of Canada (TOSCA). *Circulation* 1999; **100**:236–42.

2. Hoher M, Wohrle J, Grebe OC et al. A randomized trial of elective stenting after balloon recanalization of chronic total occlusions. *J Am Coll Cardiol* 1999; **34**:722–9.

3. Rubartelli P, Niccoli L, Verna E et al. Stent implantation versus balloon angioplasty in chronic coronary occlusions: results from the GISSOC trial. Gruppo Italiano di Studio sullo Stent nelle Occlusioni Coronariche. *J Am Coll Cardiol* 1998; **32**:90–6.

4. Sirnes PA, Golf S, Myreng Y et al. Stenting in Chronic Coronary Occlusion (SICCO): a randomized, controlled trial of adding stent implantation after successful angioplasty. *J Am Coll Cardiol* 1996; **28**:1444–51.

5. Teirstein PS, Massullo V, Jani S et al. Catheter-based radiotherapy to inhibit restenosis after coronary stenting. *N Engl J Med* 1997; **336**:1697–703.

6. Costa MA, Sabat M, van der Giessen WJ et al. Late coronary occlusion after intracoronary brachytherapy. *Circulation* 1999; **100**:789–92.

Case 42

Bifurcation In-Stent Restenosis With a Jailed Left Anterior Descending (LAD) Artery

Niall A Herity and Alan C Yeung

Background

An 81-year-old male was admitted with rapidly progressive angina. He had undergone primary angioplasty for acute myocardial infarction (AMI) 5 months before, which was his first presentation with coronary artery disease. At that time, the LAD artery and a large second diagonal branch (D2) were totally occluded and balloon angioplasty was performed, followed by stenting of the mid-LAD (S670, AVE 3.0 × 18 mm; Medtronic AVE, Santa Rosa, CA) into D2, which was thought to be larger than the distal LAD at that time. He made an uneventful recovery and had been well until c. 2 weeks before readmission, when angina recurred and progressed quickly to the stage of rest symptoms, despite appropriate medical therapy.

Angiographic commentary

Diagnostic coronary angiography was performed through the right femoral artery. An anteroposterior view with steep cranial angulation (Fig. 42.1) showed severe restenosis along the entire stent length, involving the jailed LAD which was a large artery. The right coronary artery (RCA) was dominant and normal, and the circumflex (Cx) was normal.

Femoral venous access was achieved for back-up packing if required. An 8 French (Fr) XB 4.5 guiding catheter engaged the left coronary artery (LCA) and an 0.009 inch Rotafloppy wire (Scimed, Maple Grove, MN) was advanced to the distal LAD across the stent struts. Using a 1.75 mm Rotablator burr (Scimed), six passes were made at up to 150 000 rpm. Initially, no attempt was made to cross the stent struts until satisfactory

231

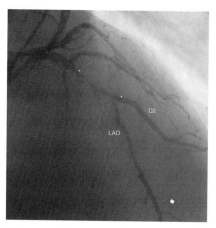

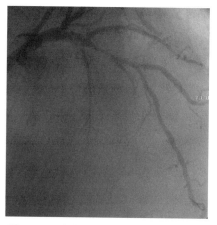

Figure 42.1. *Diagnostic coronary angiogram performed in the anteroposterior view with cranial angulation. The margins of the previously implanted S670 stent are shown by the arrows. There is diffuse restenosis along the stent associated with severe stenosis in the jailed LAD.*

Figure 42.2. *After six passes of a 1.75 mm Rotablator burr within the stent and across the struts into the distal LAD, the angiographic appearance is improved but not optimal.*

debulking was achieved inside the stent. During later passes the burr was advanced across the stent struts using the typical 'pecking' action to ensure maximal ablation of the stent and restenotic tissue before advancing the burr to the distal LAD. Using this technique there was minimal resistance to the passage of the burr, both forwards and backwards, across the stent struts. The post-rotational atherectomy result is shown in Fig. 42.2.

A second guidewire (Balance Middleweight; Guidant, Santa Clara, CA) was placed in D2 and a series of balloon inflations were performed within the stent, including kissing inflations, involving D2 and the distal LAD (Adante; Scimed; 2.5 × 20 mm balloon in each branch).

Intravascular ultrasound (IVUS) (3.2 Fr Ultracross; Scimed) revealed a significant residual plaque burden in the LAD, both distal and proximal to the S670 stent, and a decision was made to stent both ends. Following withdrawal of the diagonal guidewire, a 2.5 × 18 mm S660 stent (AVE; Medtronic) was deployed in the distal LAD, overlapping the S670 stent in a culotte fashion (Fig. 42.3).The diagonal wire was repositioned and postdilation was performed into the diagonal branch, to open up the side struts of the S660 stent.

232

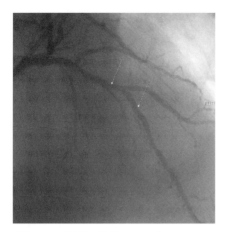

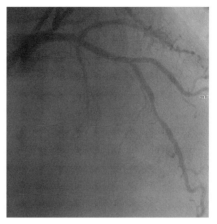

Figure 42.3. *Following the placement of a 2.5 × 18 mm S660 stent (margins indicated by the arrows), overlapping with the previously implanted S670 stent and extending into the distal LAD.*

Figure 42.4. *Final angiographic appearance following placement of a 3.0 × 12 mm NIR stent beginning just distal to D1 and overlapping the proximal end of the S670 stent.*

Finally, a 3.0 × 12 mm NIR stent (Scimed) was deployed in the mid-LAD overlapping the proximal end of the S670 stent. A repeat IVUS pullback from the distal LAD showed satisfactory stent apposition. The final angiographic result is shown in Fig. 42.4.

Discussion

Therapeutic options for this patient were either coronary artery bypass surgery (CABG) or percutaneous coronary intervention (PCI). In this setting of first restenosis confined to a single coronary arterial territory (the LAD and its branches), we typically prefer PCI over CABG if PCI is technically feasible.

In our experience, the scenario described in the present bifurcation case is not uncommon, but typically the jailed vessel is the branch rather than the parent vessel. The reverse situation encountered here made the case more challenging, in that it was necessary to achieve an excellent and stable angiographic result in the LAD, despite the fact that its distal part was jailed by stent struts which might not allow other devices to cross. We had questions that PCI was technically feasible but, after some discussion, including with the patient, proceeded to an *ad hoc* coronary intervention.

233

The device options for bifurcation in in-stent restenosis, where an important vessel is jailed, are limited to balloon angioplasty and high-speed rotational atherectomy (HSRA), with or without adjunctive brachytherapy or stent placement (but not both). We decided that balloon angioplasty alone was highly unlikely to achieve an acceptable result and therefore opted for a strategy of HSRA, adjunctive balloon angioplasty and provisional stenting. The anticipated benefits of HSRA in this setting were debulking and the ability to create a track through the side of the stent (including ablation of stent material) for future device deployment if necessary. We did not anticipate that it would provide any advantage in terms of restenosis risk or modification of vessel compliance. In selecting HSRA we sacrificed the facility for a double-wire procedure at the start of the case, although we established double-wire access as soon as it was appropriate.

Crossing stent struts with a Rotablator burr has previously been described.[1] Given that diamond is harder than stainless steel, there is no reason that the burr should not cross relatively easily. However, it is important to note that the burr only cuts in the forward direction and therefore it should not be advanced across the struts until the operator believes that the stent material has been adequately ablated and polished, so that removal of the burr is ensured.

Finally, we used the culotte technique to appose the distal LAD stent with the pre-existing S670 stent. This is only one of several stenting techniques to approach a coronary bifurcation, but it is known to be highly feasible and safe with good short-term clinical results.[2] The culotte technique has the theoretical advantage of leaving no area of vessel wall unstented at the bifurcation, and perhaps has an advantage in restenosis risk.

References

1. Morocutti G, Vendrametto F, Spedicato L et al. Bail-out rotational atherectomy to ablate stent struts after treatment of a LAD bifurcation lesion with the Trousers technique. *Cathet Cardiovasc Intervent* 2000; **50**:346–8.

2. Chevalier B, Glatt B, Royer T, Guyon P. Placement of coronary stents in bifurcation lesions by the 'culotte' technique. *Am J Cardiol* 1998; **82**:943–9.

Case 43
MANAGEMENT OF IN-STENT RESTENOSIS OF FALSE LUMEN STENTING

Aaron Wong, Soo-Teik Lim and Yean-Leng Lim

Background

A 48-year-old Chinese male, with cardiovascular risk factors of hypertension, type 2 diabetes mellitus and hyperlipidaemia, was admitted in 1997 with symptoms of exertional dyspnoea. Clinical examination showed no signs of heart failure, and there was mild inferior and lateral T-wave inversion on the electrocardiogram (ECG). Echo cardiography also showed a normal left ventricular (LV) ejection fraction (EF). A nuclear myocardial perfusion scan revealed a reversible perfusion defect in the inferolateral region. He underwent coronary angiography and, subsequently, several percutaneous coronary interventions (PCI).

Angiographic commentary

Coronary angiography in 1998 showed a short total occlusion of the right coronary artery (RCA) at the mid segment, with bridging collaterals from the proximal artery (Fig. 43.1). The left coronary system was essentially normal.

The first PCI was performed at the 1998 Singapore LIVE course to demonstrate the use of a laser wire to cross a chronic total occlusion (CTO). A Spectranetics 0.018 inch excimer laser wire and several other wires were used, but they were unable to cross the lesion and seemed to pass subintimally (Fig. 43.2a). The lesion was eventually crossed, after 2 hours, with a Shinobi 0.014 inch wire. However, there was no distal flow observed after dilatation with Maxxum 2.0 mm and Goldie 3.0 mm balloons (Figs. 43.2b and c). After verification of the guidewire position in the true lumen using distal contrast administration via a Rapid Transit Catheter (Fig. 43.2d), repeat balloon dilatation was performed with a Goldie 3.0 mm balloon. Flow was eventually established in the vessel but a long dissection

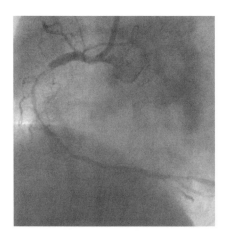

Figure 43.1. Coronary angiography of the RCA showing the pre-interventional CTO at the mid segment, with bridging collaterals opacifying the distal artery.

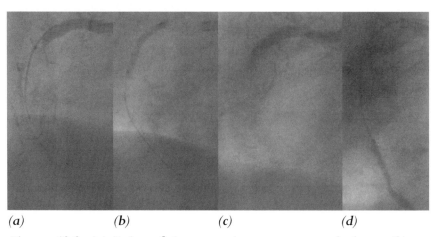

(a)   *(b)*   *(c)*   *(d)*

Figure 43.2. (a) Failure of the excimer laser wire to cross the lesion. (b) After crossing with another wire, the lesion was crossed and dilated with 2 and 3 mm balloons. (c) No distal flow was noted after dilatation. (d) Confirmation of the wire position with contrast injection opacifying the distal artery through a rapid-transit catheter.

was noted from the proximal to the mid segment of the RCA (Fig. 43.3). The dissection was stented with NIR Primo 3.0 × 32 mm and 3.0 × 25 mm stents (Figs 43.4a–c). The angiographic results were excellent, but right ventricular (RV) branches were occluded (Fig. 43.d).

The patient was well for 2 years but developed similar symptoms in February 2000, and a nuclear myocardial perfusion scan showed reversible apical, inferior and inferolateral ischaemia. Cardiac catheterization showed minor left coronary artery disease (LCA) and mid-RCA 95% long in-stent

Figure 43.3. Long dissection from the proximal to the distal RCA, noted after repeated dilatation with a 3 mm balloon.

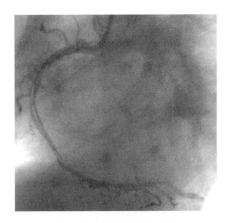

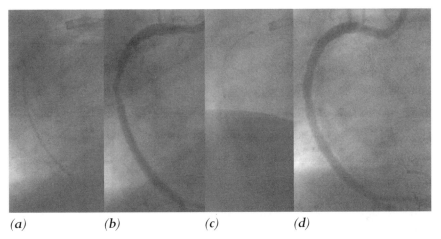

(a) *(b)* *(c)* *(d)*

Figure 43.4. (a)–(c) Two long stents were inserted to cover the dissection; (d) final angiographic picture showing occlusion of the RV branch.

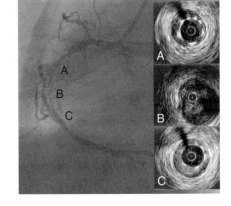

Figure 43.5. In-stent restenosis at the mid-RCA 2 years later. The IVUS showed a gap (B) between the two initial undersized stents (A and C).

237

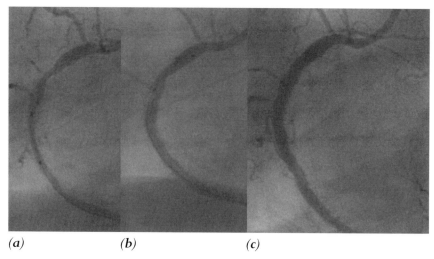

(a)   *(b)*   *(c)*

Figure 43.6. *Two short stents were inserted separately at* **(a)** *and* **(b)** *the mid-RCA to cover the gap and the proximal RCA within the previous stent.* **(c)** *Final angiographic results after optimal high-pressure post-dilatation under IVUS guidance.*

restenosis with collaterals from the LAD (Fig. 43.5). Intravascular ultrasound (IVUS) performed after a 2.5 mm balloon predilatation showed a 2 mm gap between the two NIR stents and a reference vessel diameter of 4.0 mm (Fig. 43.5). The gap was covered with an AVE S670 3.5 × 12 mm stent. The proximal RCA was further stented with an AVE S670 4.0 × 15 mm stent (Figs 43.6a and b). The final results were satisfactory both angiographically and sonographically (Fig. 43.6c).

However, 5 months later the patient had recurrent ischaemia and was admitted for unstable angina. A repeat coronary angiography showed a focal in-stent restenosis of 80% and a double-lumen appearance in the mid-RCA. Retrograde flow was also noted in the previously occluded RV branch (Fig. 43.7). IVUS showed the presence of another expansile crescent-shaped lumen outside the stent. Both lumens were within the confines of an external elastic membrane (EEM) (Fig. 43.7). It was then realized that the stents were deployed in the false lumen at the index procedure. The in-stent restenotic segment was treated with dilatation using a 3.5 × 10 mm IVT cutting balloon in the false lumen, with an acceptable outcome (Fig. 43.8).

Four months later the patient was readmitted twice for symptoms of unstable angina, and repeat cardiac catheterizaton in December 2000 showed recurrent mid-RCA in-stent restenosis with a similar double-lumen

238

appearance (Fig. 43.9). He was listed for intracoronary radiation therapy at the 2001 Singapore LIVE demonstration course. IVUS again demonstrated the dual lumen with heavy in-stent intimal proliferation at the restenotic site. The lesion was predilated with an IVT 3.5 × 10 mm cutting balloon and irradiated with a 32-P isotope using the Galileo Intravascular Radiation System (Guidant Corp.) at 20 Gray (Figs. 43.10a–c).

The patient presented again 9 months later with symptoms of angina on exertion. However, cardiac catheterization showed a patent double-lumen RCA with no recurrent in-stent restenosis (Fig. 43.11). There appeared to be no late loss during the interim from the intracoronary radiation therapy. There was slow flow noted in the RV branch, which could be the cause of the angina symptoms.

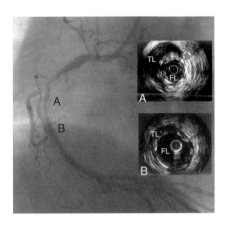

Figure 43.7. *Recurrent in-stent restenosis at the mid-RCA with IVUS (A) and (B) showing the true (TL) and false lumens (FL). There was also retrograde filling of the RV branch from the true lumen.*

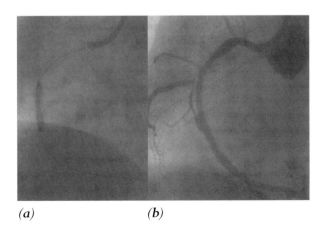

(a)   *(b)*

Figure 43.8. *(a) A cutting balloon was used for the second recurrence of in-stent restenosis with an acceptable angiographic result (b).*

239

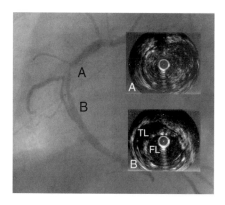

Figure 43.9. Third recurrence of in-stent restenosis (A) with a similar double-lumen appearance at the mid-RCA, with a patent RV branch. True and false lumens are clearly visible on the IVUS (B) images.

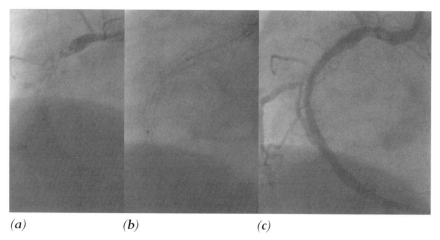

(a)   *(b)*   *(c)*

Figure 43.10. (a) Contrast injection with a spiral centring catheter (Galileo Intravascular Radiation System), inflated showing minimal distal flow. (b) Positioning of the 32-P source wire within the centring catheter. Satisfactory angiographic results post-brachytherapy.

Discussion

The success rate for opening a CTO is between 60 and 70%[1–3] and, although the restenosis rate still remains high, coronary stenting has been shown to improve the long-term patency of CTO after PCI.[4] One of the common complications of recanalizing a total occlusion, besides failure to cross the lesion, is subintimal passage of the guidewire, which can lead to failure of the procedure. But, if the guidewire re-enters the true lumen shortly after exiting it, this complication may go unnoticed, as dissections are common after balloon angioplasty in tight lesions. Without IVUS, it is difficult to differentiate between the dissection and the false lumen angiographically, and almost impossible after near-perfect reconstruction of the vessel with coronary stents. However, when the length of the subintimal passage of the guidewire is long, a longer false lumen can be created. Stenting of this false lumen will obliterate the true lumen and reconstruct another conduit for the vessel. Whether stenting in a long false lumen will increase the rate of restenosis is unclear. Another potential complication of false lumen stenting is rupture of the vessel if the guidewire is too close to the adventitial border.

There are several reported cases of intentional stenting of false lumen under IVUS guidance. Werner et al[5] reported three cases of subintimal passage of the guidewire, which later re-entered the true lumen in the RCA. Entrance and exit points into the subintima were identified on IVUS and stents deployed after confirming that the guidewire was within the adventitial border. Angiographic and clinical results were excellent. Reimers et al[6] reported a similar case, in which stents were deployed in the subintimal space of the LAD. Another case of false lumen stenting, reported by Krivonyak and Warren[7] was discovered at repeat coronary angiography 2 months later in the RCA. In all of these cases, IVUS was crucial in differentiating between the true and the false lumen, and subsequent management. The RCA seems to be more prone to subintimal dissection than the other coronary arteries,[3] the reason for which is unknown.

In our case, although the total occlusion appeared to be short, great difficulty was encountered in crossing the lesion. The guidewire went subintimal and re-entered the true lumen (Fig. 43.12a), as confirmed by contrast injection through the balloon catheter, which opacified the distal artery (Fig. 43.2d). After balloon dilatation, a long false lumen was created, which initially was thought to be a long dissection (Fig. 43.12b). The final angiographic result after stenting left no hint that the stents were in the false lumen. The undersized stents may not have obliterated the true lumen (even after dilatation with larger balloon in subsequent PCI) and continuous slow or vascular remodelling in the true lumen may have caused vessel dilatation, leading to a saccular or aneurysmal appearance (Figs 43.9 and 43.12c).[8]

Subintimal passage of the guidewire occurs in 10–20% of cases in total occlusions.[9] False lumen stenting is definitely underreported, as not all cases of total occlusion are done under IVUS guidance and can go unnoticed. As

241

Figure 43.11. Coronary angiography 9 months after brachytherapy showed no late luminal loss but there was TIMI grade 2 flow in the RV branch, which may account for the patient's anginal symptoms.

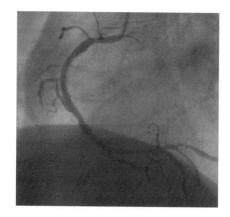

Figure 43.12. Diagramatic illustration of false lumen stenting. (**a**) Subintimal passage of the guidewire and re-entry to the true lumen. (**b**) A false lumen was created after balloon dilatation in the false lumen, which appeared like a large dissection flap. (**c**) Stenting of the false lumen initially obliterated the true lumen, which eventually recanalized, possibly through a connection between the two lumens distal to the stents.

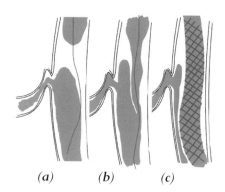

(**a**)   (**b**)   (**c**)

there were only a handful of cases of false lumen stenting reported in the literature, the management of restenosis of false lumen stenting in CTO with identifiable false lumen is unknown. The only case reported was managed by crossing and stenting the true lumen, recanalizing the true lumen by compressing the stent in the false lumen.[7] There is potential risk of rupturing the vessel.

In our case, the RCA was covered with four stents from the proximal to the mid segment, and to find the proximal entrance of the almost obliterated true lumen, which would have required crossing the stent struts as well as the neointima tissue, proved impossible. Therefore, the decision made was to establish adequate flow in the RCA by treating the in-stent restenosis in the false lumen. To our knowledge, this is only the second reported case of in-stent restenosis in the false lumen and the first case using intracoronary radiation therapy (ICRT) in the treatment of in-stent restenosis after stenting of the false lumen.

242

This case also illustrates the evolution of interventional strategies in treating in-stent restenosis. The gap between the initial two stents and the undersized stents were both factors thought to contribute to in-stent restenosis,[9] and were corrected by covering the gap with a new stent and re-expanding the stents with a larger balloon on the second PCI, with IVUS guidance. A focal in-stent restenosis lesion at the third PCI was treated with a cutting balloon, which has been shown to reduce the incidence of this event.[10] On the fourth PCI, the in-stent restenosis was treated with ICRT, using a 32-P isotope, and there was no recurrence at 9 months on angiography. Currently, trials are ongoing to see if drug-eluting stents may be the next strategy for treating in-stent restenosis.

In conclusion, stenting false lumen created by the subintimal passage of guidewires is safe provided that the guidewire re-enters the true lumen and the procedure is performed under IVUS guidance. In this situation, optimal management of in-stent restenosis of false lumen stenting is still uncertain. It appears that recanalizing the false lumen is simpler than stenting the true lumen. As in this case, using ICRT to treat in-stent restenosis in the false lumen does not appear to have created the late complication of false aneurysm formation or increased the chances of restenosis.

References

1. Melchior JP, Meier B, Urban P et al. Percutaneous transluminal coronary angioplasty for chronic total occlusion. *Am J Cardiol* 1987; **59**:535–8.

2. Stone GW, Rutherford BD, McConahay DR et al. Procedural outcome of angioplasty for total coronary artery occlusion: an analysis of 971 lesion in 905 patients. *J Am Coll Cardiol* 1990; **15**:849–56.

3. Stewart JT, Denne L, Bowker TJ et al. Percutaneous transluminal coronary angioplasty in chronic coronary artery occlusion. *J Am Coll Cardiol* 1993; 21:1371–6.

4. Sirnes A, Golf S, Myreng Y et al. Stenting in Chronic Coronary Occlusion (SICCO): a randomised, controlled trial of adding stent implantation after successful angioplasty. *J Am Coll Cardiol* 1996; 28:1444–51.

5. Werner GS, Diedrich J, Scholz K-H et al. Vessel reconstruction in total coronary occlusion with a long subintimal wire pathway: use of multiple stents under guidance of intravascular ultrasound. *Cathet Cardiovasc Intervent* 1997; **40**:46–51.

6. Reimers B, Di Mario C, Colombo A. A subintimal stent implantation for the treatment of a chronic coronary occlusion. *G Ital Cardiol* 1997; **27**:1158–63.

7. Krivonyak GS, Warren SG. Compression of a subintimal or false lumen stent by stenting in the true lumen. *J Invasive Cardiol* 2001; **13**:698–701.

8. Alfonso F, Hernandez R, Goicolea J et al. Coronary stenting for acute coronary dissection after coronary angioplasty: implications of residual dissection. *J Am Coll Cardiol* 1994; **24**:989–95.

9. Kasaoka S, Tobis JM, Akiyama T et al. Angiographic and intravascular ultrasound predictors of in-stent restenosis. *J Am Coll Cardiol* 1998; **32**:1630–5.

10. Adamian M, Colombo A, Briguori C et al. Cutting balloon angioplasty for the treatment of in-stent restenosis: a matched comparison with rotational atherectomy, additional stent implantation and balloon angioplasty. *J Am Coll Cardiol* 2001; **38**:672–9.

Case 44

COMPLEX LEFT ANTERIOR DESCENDING (LAD) ARTERY–DIAGONAL BRANCH BIFURCATION IN UNSTABLE ANGINA

Thierry Lefèvre

Background

A 71-year-old male was admitted for unstable angina. He was a current smoker but had no other cardiovascular risk factors. An electrocardiogram (ECG) showed a negative T-wave in the anterior leads. He had no creatine kinase (CK) elevation but troponine was significantly increased.

The patient was treated with heparin, nitrates, beta-blockers, aspirin and ReoPro.

A coronary angiogram showed a tight and inhomogeneous stenosis of the LAD–diagonal branch bifurcation (Fig. 44.1).

The patient was sent to our institution for percutaneous transluminal coronary angioplasty (PTCA).

Angiographic commentary

This is a true bifurcation lesion (type 1 lesion in our classification – the disease involving all limbs of the bifurcation). Because the patient had *de novo* unstable angina, we suspected the presence of thrombus and perhaps a very soft plaque.

Strategy

We decided to use direct stenting of the LAD with a wire in both branches (jailed-wire technique) to avoid distal embolization and subsequent slow flow or no-reflow.

245

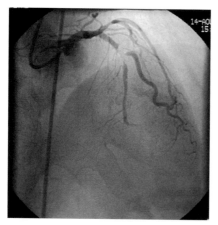

Figure 44.1.

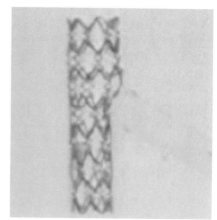

Figure 44.2.

Because the diagonal lesion was purely ostial, we planned to use only one stent in the main LAD branch, with the ostium of the side branch supported by this stent after opening the strut of the stent (Fig. 44.2).

Strategy

An extra back-up 4, 6 French (Fr) stent was used (Medtronic Zuma). The first wire (0.014 inch BMW; Guidant) was inserted into the diagonal branch (the most difficult) and the second one into the LAD (Fig. 44.3).

A Bx Velocity stent (18 × 3.5 mm; Cordis) was deployed without predilatation at 12 atmospheres (Figs 44.4 and 44.5). The angiogram showed an acceptable result, with TIMI grade 3 flow in the LAD and a subtotal stenosis of the diagonal branch at the ostium level (Fig. 44.5).

The wire was removed from the LAD and passed into the diagonal branch. Then the jailed diagonal wire was removed and passed into the LAD. The side of the stent was opened into the diagonal branch using a 3 mm Viva (Boston) balloon at 12 atmospheres (Fig. 44.6). A kissing-balloon inflation technique (Viva; Boston) was performed using a 3 mm balloon at 12 atmospheres in the diagonal branch and a 3.5 mm balloon at 10 atmospheres in the LAD (Fig. 44.7).

The final result was good (Figs 44.8 and 44.9). The CK level at 12 hours was 140 IU.

246

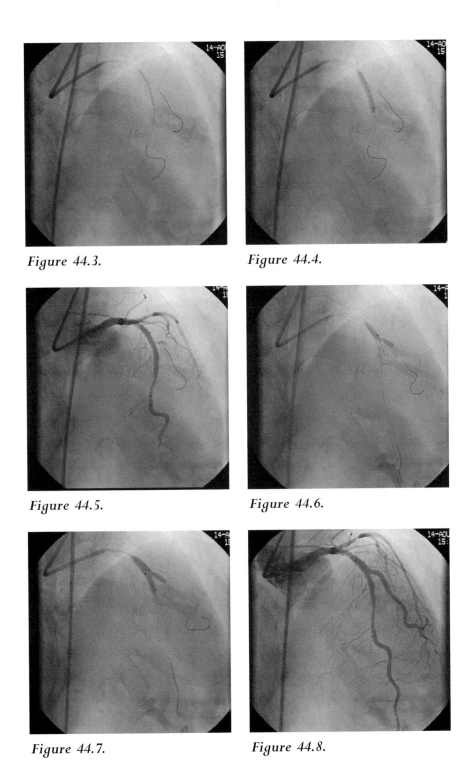

Figure 44.3.

Figure 44.4.

Figure 44.5.

Figure 44.6.

Figure 44.7.

Figure 44.8.

247

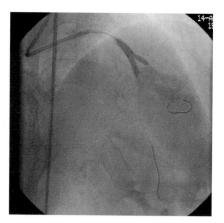

Figure 44.9.

Further reading

Lefèvre T, Louvard Y, Morice MC et al. Stenting of bifurcation lesions: classification, treatments, and results. *Cathet Cardiovasc Intervent* 2000; **49**:274–83.

Loubeyre C, Lefèvre T, Morice MC et al. Direct stenting in acute myocardial infarction. Preliminary results of a randomized study. *Circulation* 2000 (abstract).

Case 45

COMPLEX CATHETER-BASED TREATMENT: CORONARY AND CAROTID STENTING, AND MITRAL BALLOON VALVULOPLASTY

Thomas A Ischinger

Background

An 84-year-old male patient was admitted to the hospital due to a recent increase in exertional dyspnea and, more recently, dyspnea at rest (NYHA IV), and angina pectoris and occasional dizziness. The patient was known to have: calcified mitral valve stenosis, with mitral valve insufficiency grade 1–2; a VVI pacemaker implanted for atrial fibrillation (AF) (in 1991); non-insulin dependent diabetes mellitus; renal insufficiency.

Diagnostics

Cardiac catheterization was performed for re-evaluation of the situation in view of potential valve replacement surgery, despite the very reduced general condition.

Ultrasound re-examination of the carotids revealed a new ulcerated 65% diameter stenosis of the proximal right internal carotid artery (ICA), with high-grade stenosis of the origin of the external carotid. Since specific right hemispheric neurological signs attributable to the ICA stenosis had not been reported, and were not found upon neurological examination, the ICA stenosis was considered to be asymptomatic.

Cardiac catheterization, and coronary and carotid angiograms showed: high-grade bifurcational stenosis of the proximal circumflex (Cx) artery and the large marginal branch (Fig. 45.1a) [and diffuse moderate disease in the left descending anterior (LAD) artery and the right coronary artery (RCA)]; significant calcific mitral valve stenosis; [gradient 20 mmHg; mitral valve area (MVA) 1 cm^2]; mitral valve insufficiency of angiographic grade 1; preserved left ventricular (LV) function; and long, ulcerated and eccentric moderate stenosis of the proximal right ICA (Fig. 45.2a). The coronary and valvular disease represented indications for a coronary artery bypass graft (CABG) and mitral valve replacement. However, with respect to comorbidity, the cardiovascular surgeons did not recommend surgery.

Treatment and rationale

The patient was considered to be at very high risk for coronary and valvular surgery, and to have an indication for intervention for the ICA stenosis, in view of the planned coronary and valvular interventions. Consensus was reached between cardiologists, cardiovascular surgeons and neurologists that the patient should be treated by catheter intervention for coronary, carotid and mitral valve disease, rather than by surgery.

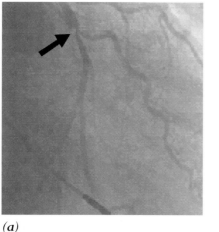

(a)

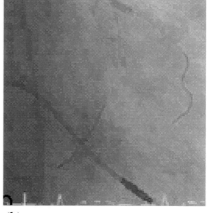

(b)

(c)

Figure 45.1. (*a*) High-grade bifurcational stenosis in LCx/marginal branch (arrow) pretreatment. (*b*) Stent implantation into the origin of the marginal branch through meshes of the LCx stent. (*c*) Result of bifurcational stenting (stents in the LCx and in the origin of the marginal branch) (arrow).

250

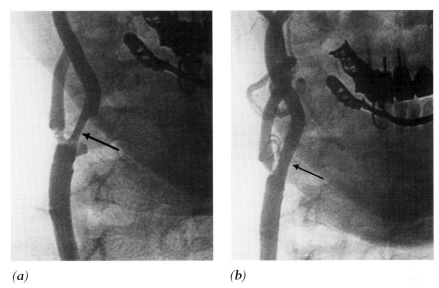

(a)   *(b)*

Figure 45.2. *(a) Moderate ulcerated long stenosis in the proximal ICA (arrow) and high-grade stenosis at take-off of external carotid pre-stent implantation. (b) After stent implantation and post-stent dilatation of the ICA. Increase of stenosis at the origin of the external carotid artery (jailed).*

Procedure

Coronary stenting

First, coronary balloon angioplasty (CBA) was performed for the bifurcational stenosis in the left Cx (LCx) artery, followed by balloon dilatation of the obtuse marginal branch (OMB) using a FL4 [6 French (Fr)] guide catheter and a 2.5 × 20 mm balloon (two wires) (Fig. 45.1b). After implantation of a 3.0 × 12 mm Nexus II stent in the LCx (across the origin of the marginal branch, with the wire left in the marginal branch), the 0.014 inch wire from the LCx was introduced through the meshes of the Nexus stent following the (roadmapping) wire into the marginal branch and a 3.0 × 12 mm AVE S670 stent advanced over it, and (after removal of the roadmapping wire) it was implanted in the stenotic origin of the marginal branch, with an excellent final result (Fig. 45.1c). Medication: pretreatment with clopidogrel 75 mg and aspirin 100 mg (both continued after the procedure), weight-adjusted heparinization [unfractionated heparin (UFH)] and, just prior to stent implantation, a weight-adjusted bolus of eptifibatide (Integrilin), followed by a 24-hour infusion and a Heparin (UFH) infusion of 15 000 IU/day for 10 days (AF) until carotid stenting was performed.

251

Carotid stenting

After a control angiogram at 10 days, confirming the very satisfactory result of the bifurcational stenting and the patient being asymptomatic from his coronary disease, a selective angiogram of the right ICA was performed using a 125 cm long FR4 Judkins catheter (5 Fr; Cordis) inside a 100 cm long multipurpose guiding catheter (7 Fr; Cordis) the latter then being advanced over the 5 Fr catheter and a 0.035 inch guidewire to an area just proximal to the carotid bifurcation. Direct stenting (DS) with a 7.0 × 30 mm Carotid Wallstent was performed, bridging the external carotid. Finally, the stent was dilated with a 5.0 × 20 mm OCCAM balloon, with a very satisfactory final result in the ICA and an increase in stenosis in the external carotid, which remained untreated (Fig. 45.2b). No protection was used, and no hemodynamic or neurological complications occurred. The patient was pretreated with clopidogrel and aspirin, and received a bolus of eptifibatide after the carotid angiogram was taken, in addition to weight-adjusted UFH. Doppler/Duplex control at 2 days confirmed good initial results. In the hours after the carotid procedure, the patient developed thrombocytopenia with a drop in the platelet count from 228 000 to 15 000. Blood tests were consistent with Heparin induced thrombo-cytopenia (HIT) type II and were positive for autoantibodies against PF4 and glycoprotein Ia/IIb. Within 1 week (clopidogrel and aspirin continued, no heparins) the platelet count normalized without further measures or complications.

Mitral balloon valvuloplasty

Two weeks later, mitral balloon valvuloplasty was carried out using a 30 mm Inoue balloon (Fig. 45.3). The gradient was reduced from 19 mmHg pre-valvuloplasty to 8 mmHg post-valvuloplasty (Figs 45.4a and b); the MVA increased from 1.0 to 2.1 cm^2. Mitral valve insufficiency increased to grade 2. No complications occurred; the patient experienced a significant relief of symptoms during follow-up and was considered to be in NYHA II.

Commentary

This case illustrates a complex minimal invasive cardiovascular catheter intervention in an aged high-risk patient with significant comorbidity, who was declined by the cardiovascular surgeons. For such patients, catheter-based treatment options may represent a valid alternative, if not the only therapeutic option. The poor renal function and consequential limited

Figure 45.3. *Inoue balloon during dilatation of calcific mitral valve (permanent pacemaker lead and pigtail catheter also visible).*

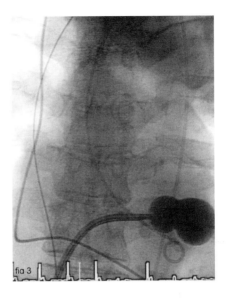

contrast tolerance of our patient forced us to stage the procedure; otherwise we would have done coronary and carotid procedures in one session. Combined or staged coronary and carotid stent placements may become the treatment of choice in selected high-risk patients. Usually, we recommend the coronary procedure first, followed by the carotid intervention, in order to avoid hemodynamically-induced myocardial ischemia if a blood pressure decrease is induced by carotis sinus irritation. In our experience, the cardiac risks of carotid stenting in such complex patients appear to be greater than the neurological risks [transient ischemic attack (TIA), stroke].

In general, the asymptomatic carotid stenosis would not be considered an indication for TIA. However, in our patient, the indication for stenting was for a recently progressive and ulcerated carotid lesion, and in preparation for coronary and valvular intervention (originally surgery). Carotid stenting appears to be a safe and efficacious treatment modality in experienced hands for selected patients.[1–6] In particular, high-risk patients and patients with coexistent heart (coronary, valvular) and carotid disease, and indication for surgery, may benefit from catheter intervention.[2–6] Simultaneous carotid and coronary surgery is still associated with a considerable risk of perioperative stroke.[3,7–9]

As the risks of mitral valve replacement surgery were considered far too high, mitral valvuloplasty[10,11] was a welcome option for our patient, who refused to continue with just conservative management of the mitral valve condition, since he felt his quality of life was unacceptable due to severe dyspnea. Despite calcific mitral stenosis and pre-existing mitral valve

253

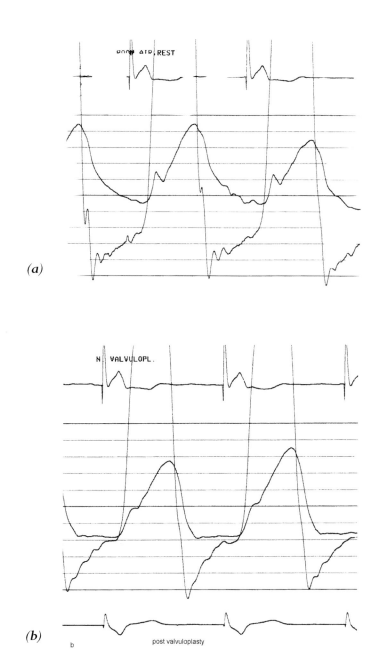

Figure 45.4. (a) *Simultaneous pressure tracings of the left ventricle and the left atrium prior to valvuloplasty.* (b) *After valvuloplasty, mitral valve gradient 8 mmHg; slight increase in V-wave, reflecting the increase in mitral valve insufficiency.*

insufficiency – which may be a contraindication if greater than angiographic grade 2 – valvuloplasty was successfully performed. Although mitral insufficiency increased after balloon dilatation, significant symptomatic relief was achieved.

Interventional pharmacology has made significant strides and, in particular, the glycoprotein IIb/IIIa antagonists have drastically reduced thrombotic complications. Even though their benefit has not been confirmed by randomized data, the glycoprotein IIb/IIIa antagonists are being used routinely in carotid stenting in our patients. The thrombocytopenia that occurred in this patient, who was receiving a second dose of eptifibatide and prolonged heparin (in combination with clopidogrel and aspirin), was rapidly reversible. The causal interrelationships (i.e. heparin and repeated doses of glycoprotein IIb/IIIa antagonists) for thrombocytopenia in this case were not fully elucidated. The findings are consistent with HIT type II, yet their interpretation is confounded by the potential of glycoprotein IIb/IIIa antagonists to trigger autoantibodies. No report on thrombocytopenia after repeated doses of eptifibatide have been published in the literature so far. There is anecdotal data to suggest that the risk of thrombocytopenia after a second administration of abciximab is causally related. The closer the first and second dates, the higher the likelihood of thrombocytopenia, with the highest incidences in the first 30 days after first administration. No clinical sequelae occurred in our case. However, we now closely follow our patients with multiple (staged) procedures, who receive complex and repeated concomitant antithrombotic treatment.

References

1. AHA advisory group. Carotid stenting and angioplasty. *Circulation* 1998; **97**:121–3.

2. Mathur A, Roubin GS, Iyer SS et al. Predictors of stroke complicating carotid artery stenting. *Circulation* 1998; **97**:1239–45.

3. Shawl FA, Efstratiou A, Hoff S et al. Combined percutaneous carotid stenting and coronary angioplasty during acute ischemic neurologic and coronary syndromes. *Am J Cardiol* 1996; **77**:1109–12.

4. Shawl F, Kadro W, Damanski M et al. Safety and efficacy of elective carotid artery stenting in high risk patients. *J Am Coll Cardiol* 2000; **35**:1721–8.

5. Ischinger TA. Carotis stent – *Pro. Z Kardiol* 2000; **89(Suppl 6)**: VI/76.

6. Ischinger TA. Carotid stenting: which stent for which lesion? *J Interven Cardiol* 2001; **14**:614–24.

255

7.   Rothwell PM. Carotid endarterectomy for recently symptomatic carotid stenosis: consistent results from two large randomized trials. *Eur Heart J* 1999; **20**:1055–7.

8.   Dashe JF, Pessin MS, Murphy RE, Payne DD. Carotid occlusive disease and stroke risk in coronary artery bypass graft surgery. *Neurology* 1997; **49**:678–86.

9.   Trachiotis GD, Pfister AJ. Management strategy for simultaneous carotid endarterectomy and coronary revascularization. *Ann Thorac Surg* 1997; **64**:1013–18.

10. Palacios I, Block P, Brandi S et al. Percutaneous balloon valvotomy for patients with severe mitral stenosis. *Circulation* 1987; **75**:778–84.

11. Jung B, Cormier B, Ducimétiere P et al. Immediate results of percutaneous mitral commissurotomy: a predictive model on a series of 1514 patients. *Circulation* 1996; **94**:2123–30.

Case 46

Stenting Of The Unprotected Left Main Coronary Artery (LMCA) And The Left Anterior Descending (LAD) And Total Right External Iliac Arteries In One Session

Talib K Majwal

Introduction

LMCA disease is found in 3–5% of patients undergoing cardiac catheterization.[1–2] Whereas medical treatment of patients with LMCA disease is associated with poor prognosis,[3] revascularization by coronary bypass surgery has been shown to improve survival[4,5] and is generally the preferred therapeutic option.

Current techniques of stent deployment, intravascular ultrasound (IVUS) guidance and new antiplatelet medications have been associated with a dramatic reduction in the risk of subacute stent thrombosis.[6–9]

However, iliac artery angioplasty represents an important skill for the cardiovascular interventionist to master, not only to relieve patient's lower extremity symptoms, but also to preserve access for what may be life-saving procedures such as coronary angioplasty or intraaortic balloon counter pulsation.

Case report

A 57-year-old male with no obvious risk factors of ischemic heart disease was referred to our center with unstable angina class IIB2.

The patient had a history of intermittent claudication at 500 m over the last year.

257

On admission, the patient had a normal electrocardiogram (ECG), apart from frequent ventricular ectopics.

Emergency coronary angiography via left femoral access (because of an absent right femoral pulse) was undertaken and demonstrated 80% stenosis of the mid- and distal LMCA, 90% of the mid-LAD B1 lesion, and normal left circumflex (LCx) and dominant right coronary (RCA) arteries. (Fig. 46.1).

Selective right common iliac angiography showed total external iliac occlusion with extensive collaterals to the distal segment. (Fig. 46.3).

After premedication (10 000 IU of heparin, 300 mg clopidogrel and 325 mg aspirin orally) the procedure was carried out using a 7 French (Fr) 3.5 Judkin left Vista BT guiding catheter (Cordis Corp., Miami Lakes, FL); a 0.014 inch Wisdom 180 cm supersoft guidewire (Cordis) crossed the LMCA into the LAD. IVUS (Vision Five-64 F/X; Endosonics Corp., Rancho Cordora, CA) was used to guide direct stenting (DS) of the LMCA with a 4.0 × 13 mm Bx Velocity stent (Cordis); post-stent dilation was performed with 5.0 mm Bypass Speedy balloon (Schneider, Minneapolis, MN). The minimal luminal diameter (MLD) after stenting was 5.1 mm and the cross-sectional area (CSA) was 16.3 mm^2 (Fig. 46.5). DS of the mid-LAD was performed with 3.0 × 16 mm JoStent Flex stent (JoMed GmbH, Rangendingen, Germany), with a good final result for both the LMCA and the LAD. (Fig. 46.4).

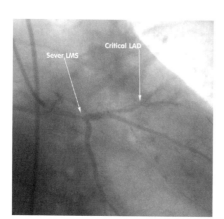

Figure 46.1. *Right anterior oblique (RAO) projection, showing severe distal left main stem coronary stenosis with a negative remodeling effect and mid-LAD stenosis.*

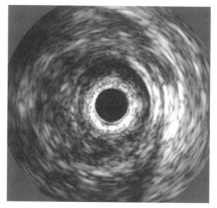

Figure 46.2. *IVUS of the distal left main stem coronary shows calcified atheroma; MLD 1.9 mm; CSA 6.2 mm^2.*

258

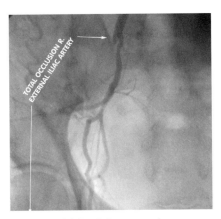

Figure 46.3. *Selective right common iliac artery angiography showing total occlusion of the right external iliac artery.*

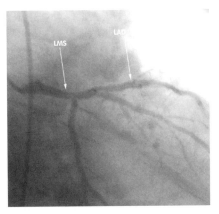

Figure 46.4. *RAO projection: a good result after stenting, showing the distal left main stem coronary and the mid-LAD.*

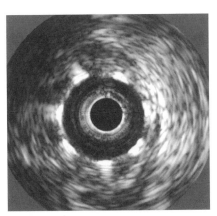

Figure 46.5. *IVUS of the distal left main stem coronary showing a well-expanded stent in the distal left main (MLD 5.1 mm CSA, 16.3 mm^2).*

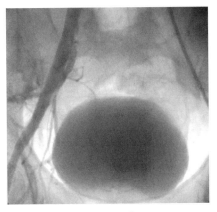

Figure 46.6. *Successful revascularization of the right external iliac artery.*

An 8 Fr RDC (renal) guiding catheter (Cordis) crossed to the right common iliac artery from the contralateral side. The total occlusion of the external iliac was crossed with a 0.35 inch Terumo wire, then DS was undertaken with a 10 × 60 mm self-expandable SMART stent (Cordis) and post-dilated with a 10 mm OPTA peripheral balloon, with a good final result (Fig. 46.6).

259

The whole procedure required 300 ml of Hexabrix 320 contrast media (Guerbet, Cedex, France); the fluoroscopy time was 17.8 minutes.

The patient was discharged well the next day, on clopidogrel 75 mg daily and aspirin 325 mg daily, and was scheduled for a 3-month follow-up angiography.

Discussion

Conventional percutaneous transluminal coronary angioplasty (PTCA), for which coronary artery bypass grafting (CABG) has been the gold-standard therapy for years, has yielded poor results in unprotected LMCA lesions. The development of coronary stents, together with new antiplatelet regimens, has improved the potency of PCI in left main disease. The incidence of restenosis warrants reappraisal of LMCA stenosis. Elective stenting of unprotected LMCA stenosis should, theoretically, provide the following advantages over balloon angioplasty: reduction of the risk of abrupt closure; greater acute gain; a lower restenosis rate at follow-up.[10]

Surgical treatment of iliac occlusion is reported to have a 74–95% 5-year patency, which is comparable to balloon angioplasty,[11] and the availability of endovascular stents has dramatically affected the results of balloon angioplasty of iliac arteries.[12–14]

This patient is patient 52 to undergo stenting of an unprotected left main stenosis in our center over the last 2 years.

Stented LMCA patients who have smaller final stent MLD and CSA, or poor left ventricular (LV) function, tend to have higher mortality than those with normal LV functions and bigger MLD and CSA.[15] Therefore, IVUS guided stenting of the LMCA is essential. With the increasing experience of the interventional cardiologist in peripheral arterial intervention and flexible new equipment, a combination of both coronary and peripheral arterial intervention in the same session will become common practice.

References

1.   Cohen MV, Cohen PF, Herman MV, Gorlin R. Diagnosis and prognosis of main left coronary artery obstruction. *Circulation* 1972; **45**:157–65.

2.   Cohen MV, Gorlin R. Left main coronary artery disease, clinical experience from 1964-1974. *Circulation* 1975; **52**:272–85.

3.   Conly MJ, Ely RL, Kissloy J et al. The prognosis spectrum of left main stenosis. *Circulation* 1978; **57**:947–52.

4.   Varnauskas E, for the European Coronary Surgery study group. Twelve years follow up of survival in the randomised European coronary study group. *N Engl J Med* 1998; **319**:332–7.

5.   The Veterans Administration coronary artery bypass surgery cooperative group. Eleven years survival in the veteran's administration randomised trial of coronary bypass surgery for stable angina. *N Engl J Med* 1984; **311**:1333–9.

6.   Colombo A, Hall P, Nakamura S et al. Intra-coronary stenting without anti-coagulation accomplished with intravascular ultrasound guidance. *Circulation* 1995; **41**:1676–88.

7.   Gregorini L, Marco J, Fajadet J et al. Ticlopidine and aspirin pre-treatment reduce coagulation and platelet activation during coronary dilation procedure. *J Am Coll Cardiol* 1997; **29**:13–20.

8.   Park SJ, Park SW, Hong MK et al. Stenting of unprotected left main coronary artery stenosis: immediate and late outcome. *J Am Coll Cardiol* 1998; **31**:37–42.

9.   Schomig A, Neumann FJ, Kastrats A. A randomised comparison of antiplatelet and anticoagulation therapy after placement of coronary stent. *N Engl J Med* 1996; **334**:1084–9.

10. Black A, Cortina R, Bossi I et al. Unprotected left main coronary artery stenting. *J Am Coll Cardiol* 2001; **37**:832–8.

11. Johnston KW. Balloon angioplasty: predictive factors for long-term success. *Semin Vasc Surg* 1989; **3**:117–22.

12. Murphy KD, Encarnacion CE, le VA, Palmaz JC. Iliac artery stent placement with Palmaz stent: follow up study. *J Vasc Interven Radiol* 1995; **6**:321–9.

13. Sapoval MR, Chatellier G, Long AL et al. Self expandable stents for treatment of iliac artery obstructive lesions: long term success and prognostic factors. *Am J Radiol* 1996; **166**:1173–9.

14   Sullivan TM, Childs MB, Bacharch JM et al. Percutaneous transluminal angioplasty and primary stenting of the iliac arteries in 288 pt. *J Vasc Surg* 1997; **25**:824–39.

15. Bosch JL, Hunink MG. Meta-analysis of the result of percutaneous transluminal angioplasty and stent placement for aorto-iliac occlusive disease. *Radiology* 1997; **204**:87–96.

261

Case 47

Combined Carotid Artery With Total Mid-Left Anterior Descending (LAD) Artery And Circumflex (Cx) Artery Stenting In One Session

Talib K Majwal

Introduction

Carotid and coronary disease represent a difficult therapeutic dilemma. The surgical approach in such patients is associated with a high risk for stroke, myocardial infarction and mortality. Recent progress in coronary devices and peripheral equipment makes it possible to combine carotid and coronary techniques in anatomically-challenging patients.

Background

A 68-year-old male presented with a history of anterior myocardial infarction and recurrent transient ischemic attacks (TIA). He presented with recurrent anginal chest pain (Canadian cardiovascular class IV); he was a heavy smoker but had no history of hypertension or diabetes mellitus and had a normal serum lipid profile.

Clinical examination was unremarkable, apart from a left carotid bruit.

Angiography revealed total occlusion of the mid-LAD at two sites (Fig. 47.1), a critical left Cx (LCx) (Fig. 47.2) and a normal right coronary artery (RCA).

Quantitative measurements of the carotid artery revealed a 66% ulcerated stenosis at the beginning of the right internal carotid artery (Fig. 47.3). The left ventricular (LV) ejection fraction (EF) was 54%.

Our approach was to undertake carotid intervention before the coronary intervention, in order to prevent stroke in case hypotension or other complications occurred during coronary intervention.

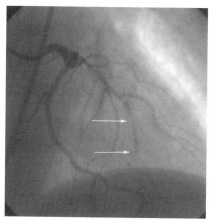

Figure 47.1. *Right anterior oblique (RAO) projection, showing total mid-LAD at two sites after DS.*

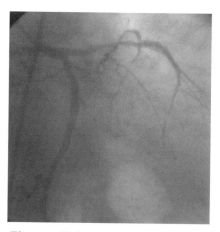

Figure 47.2. *RAO projection: critical proximal LCx.*

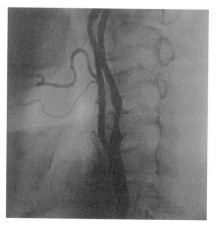

Figure 47.3. *Left internal carotid artery showing a 66% ulcerating stenosis (proximally).*

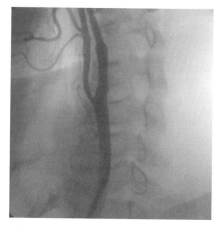

Figure 47.4. *Left internal carotid artery after stenting with an 8.0 × 16 mm stent.*

Via a 7 French (Fr) 90 cm introducer sheath, the left common carotid artery was selectively cannulated, an 8 mm Angioguard filter protection device (Cordis Corp., Miami Lakes, FL) was then passed through the lesion.

Direct stenting (DS) was undertaken with an 8.0 × 16 mm peripheral JoStent stent (JoMed GmbH, Rangendingen, Germany) inflated up to 10 atmospheres. A good result was achieved without complications (Fig. 47.4).

264

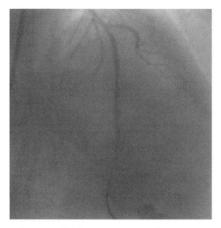

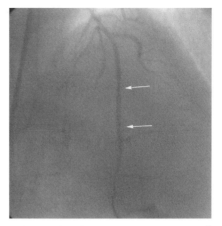

Figure 47.5. RAO cranial projection: successful revascularization of the total LAD with two stents, both 3.0 × 13 mm.

Figure 47.6. RAO projection: DS of the LCx with a 3.5 × 13 mm stent.

The LAD total occlusion was crossed by a 0.014 inch Shinobi guidewire (Cordis) and, after predilation with a 2.0 mm balloon, two 3.0 × 13 mm Bx Velocity stents (Cordis) were deployed under intravascular ultrasound (IVUS) guidance, with a good result (Fig. 47.5). This was followed by DS of the LCx lesion with a 3.5 × 13 mm Bx Velocity stent at up to 14 atmospheres, again with a good result (Fig. 47.6).

The patient was discharged well the next morning, on clopidogrel 75 mg and ASA 325 mg for 3 months.

At 6 months follow-up the patient was asymptomatic and living an active life.

With increased experience of the interventional cardiologist in peripheral and carotid arterial intervention, and flexible new equipment, a combination of coronary and other arterial interventions at the same session will become common practice.

Case 48

Beware The Calcified Circumflex (Cx)

I Patrick Kay, Alan Whelan and Gerard T Wilkins

Case

A 75-year-old female presented with unstable angina. Coronary angiography revealed a tight calcified proximal Cx artery stenosis (Fig. 48.1). A BMW guidewire was passed to the distal vessel. Passage of a 3.0 × 20 mm balloon was difficult due to extensive proximal tortuosity and calcification. Coronary balloon angioplasty (Fig. 48.2) led to a dissection propagating proximally into the left main stem (LMS) artery (Fig. 48.3). The patient remained hemodynamically stable throughout this incident. A second wire was passed to the distal left anterior descending (LAD) artery. Intravascular ultrasound (IVUS) was performed (Fig. 48.4). The proximal Cx and the LAD were stented consecutively (Figs. 48.5 and 48.6). The LMS was stented, resulting in a 'Y' stent configuration (Fig. 48.7). A kissing-balloon inflation was performed in the LMS to ensure good stent apposition (Fig. 48.8). The final angiographic appearance of the treated vessels was satisfactory (Fig. 48.9). At the 6-month clinical follow-up the patient was symptom-free and angiographic appearances were satisfactory.

Comment

The evolution of low-profile, highly trackable balloons and stents has enabled the interventional cardiologist to treat lesions that could not conceivably have been treated a few years ago. This advantage is a two-edged sword – difficult lesions such as the calcified proximal Cx can now be treated, but the complications, as seen in this case, can be horrendous. In the above case, the patient remained hemodynamically stable despite a grim angiographic appearance. This enabled the operator to image the lesion with IVUS and define the site of dissection, the severity and the axial length. In addition, it permitted an accurate choice of stent size relative to true vessel size and length. This is important for the LMS where the total vessel area is

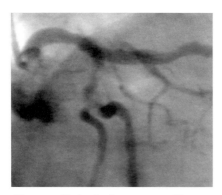

Figure 48.1. *Right anterior oblique (RAO) projection: significant lesion in a tortuous, calcified proximal Cx artery.*

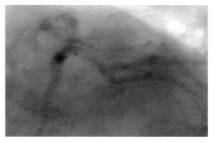

Figure 48.2. *Balloon dilatation. Note the distal tip of the balloon extends into the obtuse marginal.*

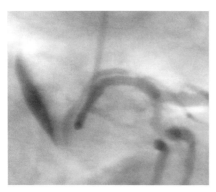

Figure 48.3. *Marked dissection propagating from the Cx into the LMS artery and aorta root. A double shadow is seen in the region of the LMS and is continuous with the aortic area of the dissection (left).*

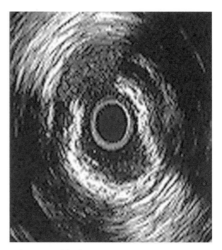

Figure 48.4. *IVUS image demonstrating a submedial dissection (10 o'clock to 1 o'clock) adjacent to an area of extensive calcification (1 o'clock to 10 o'clock). Note the absence of an echo signal deep to the calcification and reverberation inferiorly.*

frequently greater than that perceived angiographically; in this case, kissing-balloon inflation was necessary to ensure good stent apposition.

LMS dissection as a consequence of percutaneous transluminal coronary angioplasty (PTCA) is a rare and possibly underreported phenomenon. Patients are frequently stabilized on the operating table and then transferred to cardiac surgery. The above case suggests that a percutaneous approach assisted by IVUS imaging may give a satisfactory result in selected individuals.

268

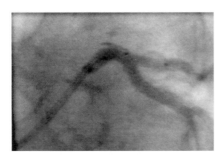

Figure 48.5. Stent implantation in the proximal LAD.

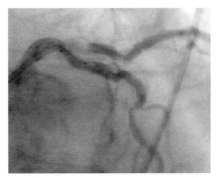

Figure 48.6. Stent implantation in the proximal Cx.

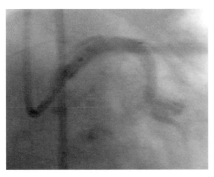

Figure 48.7. Stent implantation in the LMS.

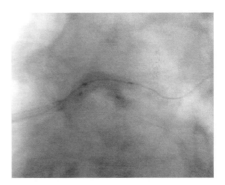

Figure 48.8. 'Kissing-balloon' inflation in the proximal LAD/Cx and in the LMS.

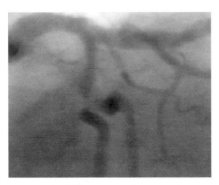

Figure 48.9. Final angiographic appearance. This closely reflects the image seen at the 6-month follow-up.

269

Case 49

ROTATIONAL ATHERECTOMY OF AN UNDEREXPANDED STENT

Yoshio Kobayashi, George Dangas, Martin B Leon and Jeffrey W Moses

Background

A 69-year-old male with a history of prior coronary artery bypass surgery with previous stent implantation in the proximal left circumflex artery (LCx) was admitted due to exertional angina.

Angiographic commentary

Coronary angiography revealed in-stent restenosis of 90% in the proximal LCx (Fig. 49.1a). The left anterior descending coronary (LAD) artery and the right coronary artery (RCA) were totally occluded. A saphenous vein graft (SVG) to the LAD had a 70% stenosis at the distal anastomosis and an SVG to the RCA had a 70% stenosis at the distal segment.

The lesions in the SVG to the LAD and RCA were successfully treated with stents. Conventional balloon angioplasty was performed to treat in-stent restenosis in the proximal LCx. Although a 3.25 mm NC Ranger balloon catheter (Boston Scientific, Maple Grove, MN) was inflated up to 25 atmospheres (Fig. 49.1b), full expansion could not be achieved (Fig. 49.1c). The intervention was terminated, but the patient remained symptomatic and was referred to our hospital for a repeat attempt at angioplasty of the lesion in the proximal LCx.

An 8 French (Fr) VL 4 guiding catheter (Boston Scientific) was engaged at the left main ostium. Coronary angiography demonstrated tandem lesions in the proximal LCx (Fig. 49.2a). Intravascular ultrasound (IVUS) imaging was performed in the proximal LCx using a 30 MHz 3.2 Fr UltraCross catheter (Boston Scientific). IVUS images revealed intimal hyperplasia at the proximal segment of the stent and stent underexpansion at the distal stent segment

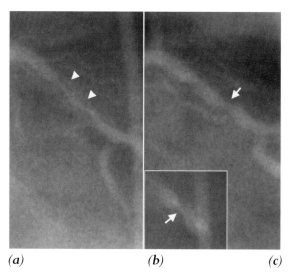

(a)   *(b)*   *(c)*

Figure 49.1. *Coronary angiography showing in-stent restenosis of 90% severity in the proximal LCx artery in the right anterior oblique (RAO) projection (arrowheads). (a) Conventional balloon angioplasty is performed with a 3.25 mm NC Ranger balloon catheter inflated to 25 atmospheres. However, the balloon catheter is not fully expanded (arrow) (b) and it is not dilatable (arrow) (c). Reprinted from Catheterization and Cardiovascular Interventions, 52, Kobayashi Y, Teirstein P, Linnemeier T, Stone G, Leon M, Moses J, Rotational atherectomy (stentablation) in a lesion with stent underexpansion due to heavily calcified plaque, 208–11, Copyright (2001), with permission from John Wiley & Sons, Inc[20] with permission.*

(Fig. 49.3a), where the lesion behind the stent struts appeared heavily calcified. Due to the previous difficulties in achieving adequate balloon expansion, rotational atherectomy was attempted after a 0.009 inch RotaWire (extra support) with a 0.014 inch tip (Boston Scientific) was placed across the lesion. The rotational speed was set at 150 000 rpm and the catheter advanced slowly in a gentle pecking motion through the lesion. A 1.5 mm burr was used initially, followed by a 1.75 mm burr. Following this initial atherectomy, angiography indicated improvement in the lumen diameter (Fig. 49.2b), but IVUS imaging still showed a small lumen size with a heavily calcified plaque behind the stent (Fig. 49.3b). Additional rotational atherectomy with a 2.0 mm burr was performed. All ablation intervals were <30 seconds and a decrease in rotational speed to >5000 rpm was not observed. A 3.0 mm Quantum Ranger balloon catheter (Boston

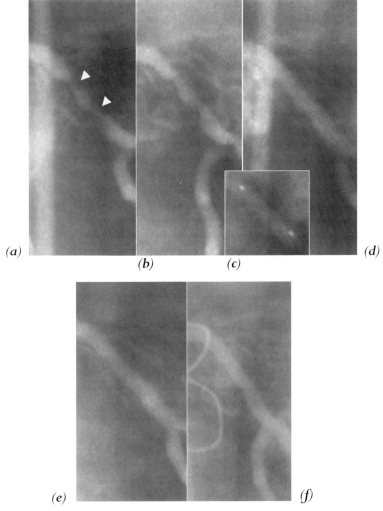

Figure 49.2. (a) Coronary angiography showing tandem lesions in the proximal LCx (arrowheads). (b) Angiogram after rotational atherectomy with a 1.75 mm burr shows improvement in lumen diameter. (c) Adjunctive balloon angioplasty with a 3.0 mm balloon catheter inflated to 12 atmospheres is performed. Note that the balloon catheter is fully expanded. (d) Angiogram demonstrating a good result. (e) After catheter-based intracoronary gamma radiation, this final angiogram shows a good result. (f) This follow-up angiogram demonstrates no restenosis. Reprinted from Catheterization and Cardiovascular Interventions, 52, Kobayashi Y, Teirstein P, Linnemeier T, Stone G, Leon M, Moses J, Rotational atherectomy (stentablation) in a lesion with stent underexpansion due to heavily calcified plaque, 208–11, Copyright (2001), with permission from John Wiley & Sons, Inc[20] with permission.

273

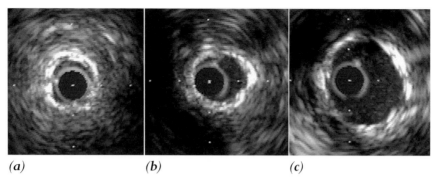

(a)   (b)   (c)

Figure 49.3. (a) IVUS image showing stent underexpansion due to 360°
circumferencially calcified plaque. (b) After rotational atherectomy with a
1.75 mm burr, this IVUS image demonstrates that there is still a small lumen
with heavily calcified plaque. (c) This final IVUS image shows a good round
lumen with absence of stent struts between 6 and 9 pm. Reprinted from
Catheterization and Cardiovascular Interventions, 52, Kobayashi Y, Teirstein
P, Linnemeier T, Stone G, Leon M, Moses J, Rotational atherectomy
(stentablation) in a lesion with stent underexpansion due to heavily calcified
plaque, 208–11, Copyright (2001), with permission from John Wiley & Sons,
Inc[20] with permission.

Scientific) was then passed through the lesion. The guidewire was then
changed to a 0.014 inch All Star guidewire (Guidant, Tamecula, CA).
The balloon catheter was pulled back to the lesion. Balloon inflation at
12 atmospheres was performed and a fully expanded balloon catheter was
observed (Fig. 49.2c). Additional balloon angioplasty with a 3.5 mm Ranger
balloon catheter (Boston Scientific) inflated to 12 atmospheres was then
performed. Angiography indicated an excellent result (Fig. 49.2d). IVUS
images revealed a round lumen and, in some regions of the stented segment,
absence of stent struts (Fig. 49.3c). A Checkmate radiation catheter (Cordis
Corp., Miami, FL) was then placed in the proximal LCx and catheter-based
intracoronary gamma radiation (14 Gray at 2 mm) was performed to prevent
recurrence of intimal hyperplasia within the stent (primarily, the proximal
area was stenosed due to intimal hyperplasia). The final angiogram
demonstrated excellent acute results (Fig. 49.2e).

With respect to adjunct pharmacological therapy, the patient received
aspirin 325 mg and clopidogrel 450 mg prior to intervention, and a 3 minute
bolus of tirofiban (10 μg/kg) was administered IV followed by an IV infusion

of 0.15 μg/kg/minute for 12 hours. Following stent implantation, daily therapy with aspirin 325 mg and clopidogrel 75 mg was continued for 12 months. After the procedure, creatine kinase (CK) myocardial band (MB) elevation was not observed and the patient's hospital course was uneventful. Subacute stent thrombosis was not observed. Follow-up angiography was performed 3 months later and revealed no recurrent restenosis (Fig. 49.2f).

Discussion

Although previous randomized trials[1] have demonstrated lower restenosis rates in selected lesions with coronary stents compared to conventional balloon angioplasty, in-stent restenosis remains an important clinical problem.[2] IVUS studies[3] have demonstrated that coronary stenting eliminates arterial remodeling. Therefore, neointimal hyperplasia is solely responsible for in-stent restenosis. However, in-stent restenosis due to stent underexpansion (pseudo in-stent restenosis) is sometimes observed.[4]

Early experiences with coronary stenting demonstrated high stent thrombosis rates.[5] Initially, stent underexpansion was considered to be one of the reasons for high subacute stent thrombosis rates.[6] To optimize stent deployment and prevent stent thrombosis, high-inflation pressure dilatation and antiplatelet therapy were introduced.[6,7] However, despite high-inflation pressure dilatation, stent underexpansion is still sometimes observed in rigid lesions such as those that are heavily calcified.[8,9] While conventional balloon angioplasty can be attempted, rigid calcified plaque may prevent full balloon expansion.

Treatment of heavily calcified coronary lesions using balloon angioplasty has been associated with reduced angiographic success and increased complications.[10,11] Rotational atherectomy has improved success rates in calcified lesions.[11,12] The Rotablator device preferentially cuts hard plaque, which changes plaque compliance, rendering the lesion more amenable to balloon dilatation.[13] Although coronary stenting eliminates elastic recoil, in heavily calcified lesions, inadequate stent expansion can occur.[8,9] To facilitate stent expansion, rotational atherectomy followed by stenting is recommended in heavily calcified lesions.[14] However, in this case, the stent had been deployed in a heavily calcified lesion, which had resulted in stent underexpansion.[8,9] Thus, to ablate the calcified plaque, ablation of stent struts was required.

In experimental in vitro and in vivo preparations, the vast majority of particulate debris generated by rotational atherectomy was sufficiently small

275

to traverse the coronary circulation without obstructing capillaries.[15,16] However, in these studies, arterial calcification and/or complex atherosclerotic plaque were not present. Previous clinical studies showed a procedural myocardial infarction rate of up to 25% with rotational atherectomy when complex, calcified plaque is treated.[14] In this case, rotational atherectomy clearly ablated calcified plaque because the vessel compliance increased, allowing full balloon expansion. This means that rotational atherectomy also ablated stent struts, producing metallic particles. There is little information regarding the possible size of such metallic particles and possible adverse clinical consequences. In this particular case, there was no slow flow during or after rotational atherectomy and no cardiac enzyme elevation was observed. Rotational atherectomy was performed with a stepped burr approach, taking care to avoid any drop in rotational speed. In addition, the platelet glycoprotein IIb/IIIa receptor inhibitor tirofiban was used for additional protection against periprocedural myocardial damage.[17]

Another possible concern about this procedure is subacute or late stent thrombosis because some stent struts may contact blood flow directly after rotational atherectomy. However, previous studies showed low subacute stent thrombosis rates after stenting following rotational atherectomy with antiplatelet therapy.[14,18] In the light of the patient's subsequent treatment with intracoronary brachytherapy and the increased risk of delayed thrombosis,[19] clopidogrel was prescribed for 12 months.

Another option to treat this lesion was coronary artery bypass surgery. However, in this case, bypass surgery was performed 6 years ago, and the SVG to the LAD and the RCA were patent.

This case shows a challenging strategy to treat a lesion with stent underexpansion due to heavily calcified plaque. Despite our success, it should be emphasized that the best strategy is to avoid inadequate stent expansion. When a calcified lesion is observed by angiography, direct stenting (DS) should be avoided and the operator should evaluate severity and location of calcification by IVUS, and pretreat with rotational atherectomy if necessary.

References

1. Fischman D, Leon MB, Baimi DS et al for the Stent Restenosis Study Investigators. A randomized comparison of coronary stent placement and balloon angioplasty in the treatment of coronary artery disease. *N Engl J Med* 1994; **331**:496–501.

2. Kobayashi Y, De Gregorio J, Kobayashi N et al. Stented segment length as an independent predictor of restenosis. *J Am Coll Cardiol* 1999; **34**:651–9.

3. Mintz GS, Popma JJ, Hong MK et al. Intravascular ultrasound to discern device-specific effects and mechanisms of restenosis. *Am J Cardiol* 1996; **78(Suppl 3A)**:18–22.

4. Mintz GS, Hoffmann R, Mehran R et al. In-stent restenosis: the Washington Hospital Center experience. *Am J Cardiol* 1998; **81**:7E–13E.

5. Nath FC, Muller DW, Ellis SG et al. Thrombosis of a flexible coil coronary stent; frequency, predictors and clinical outcome. *J Am Coll Cardiol* 1993; **21**:622–7.

6. Colombo A, Hall P, Nakamura S et al. Intracoronary stenting without anticoagulation accomplished with intravascular ultrasound guidance. *Circulation* 1995; **91**:1676–88.

7. Moussa I, Oetgen M, Roubin G et al. Effectiveness of clopidogrel and aspirin versus ticlopidine and aspirin in preventing stent thrombosis after coronary stent implantation. *Circulation* 1999; **99**:2364–6.

8. Albrecht D, Kaspers S, Fussi R et al. Coronary plaque morphology affects stent deployment: assessment by intracoronary ultrasound. *Cathet Cardiovasc Diagn* 1996; **38**:229–35.

9. Hoffmann, R, Mintz GS, Popma JJ et al. Treatment of calcified lesions with Palmaz–Schatz stents. An intravascular ultrasound study. *Eur Heart J* 1998; **19**:1224–31.

10. Detre K, Holubkov R, Kelsey S et al. Percutaneous transluminal coronary angioplasty in 1985–1986 and 1977–1981. The National Heart, Lung, and Blood Institute Registry. *N Engl J Med* 1988; **318**:265–70.

11. Brogan III WC, Popma JJ, Pichard AD et al. Rotational coronary atherectomy after unsuccessful coronary balloon angioplasty. *Am J Cardiol* 1993; **71**:794–8.

12. MacIsaac AI, Bass TA, Buchbinder M et al. High speed rotational atherectomy: outcome in calcified and noncalcified coronary artery lesions. *J Am Coll Cardiol* 1995; **26**:731–6.

13. Mintz GS, Potkin BN, Keren G et al. Intravascular ultrasound evaluation of the effect of rotational atherectomy in obstructive atherosclerotic coronary artery disease. *Circulation* 1992; **86**:1383–93.

14. Hong MK, Mintz GS, Popma JJ et al. Safety and efficacy of elective stent implantation following rotational atherectomy in large calcified coronary arteries. *Cathet Cardiovasc Diagn* 1996; **38(Suppl 3)**:50–4.

15. Hansen DD, Auth DC, Vracko R, Ritchie JL. Rotational artherectomy in atherosclerotic rabbit arteries. *Am Heart J* 1988; **115**:160–5.

277

16.   Hansen DD, Auth DC, Hall M, Ritchie JL. Rotational endarterectomy in normal canine coronary arteries: preliminary report. *J Am Coll Cardiol* 1988; **11**:1073–7.

17.   Koch KC, vom Dahl J, Kleinhans E et al. Influence of a platelet GPIIb/IIIa receptor antagonist on myocardial hyperfusion during rotational atherectomy as assessed by myocardial Tc-99m sestamibi scintigraphy. *J Am Coll Cardiol* 1999; **33**:998–1004.

18.   Kobayashi Y, De Gregorio J, Kobayashi N et al. Lower restenosis rate with stenting following aggressive versus less aggressive rotational atherectomy. *Cathet Cardiovasc Intervent* 1999; **46**:406–14.

19.   Waksman R, Bhargava B, Mintz GS et al. Late total occlusion after intracoronary brachytherapy for patients with in-stent restenosis. *J Am Coll Cardiol* 2000; **36**:65–8.

20.   Koboyashi Y, Terstein PS, Linnemeier TJ et al. Rotational atherectomy (stentablation) in a lesion with stent underexpansion due to heavily calcified plaque. *Cathet Cardiovasc Intervent* 2001; **52**(2):208–11.

278

Case 50
SPIRAL DISSECTION MANAGED CONSERVATIVELY

Peter Ruygrok

Background

A 70-year-old Chinese female with a 5-month history of increasing effort angina underwent an exercise treadmill test and managed only 3 minutes 40 seconds of the Bruce protocol, stopping because of chest pain associated with ischaemic changes. Her risk factors for coronary artery disease were a raised serum cholesterol, treated with simvastatin 20 mg (total cholesterol 4.9 mmol/l), and a history of hypertension, for which she was on felodipine 5 mg and metoprolol 47.5 mg. She also took 100 mg aspirin daily. Her resting electrocardiogram (ECG) showed that sinus rhythm and was within normal limits.

Angiographic commentary

Coronary angiography revealed mild disease in the left anterior descending (LAD) artery, a diffusely diseased mid-right coronary artery (RCA), with a total occlusion more distally and a severe focal lesion in the left circumflex (LCx) artery, which appeared suitable for percutaneous coronary interventional (PCI) treatment (Fig. 50.1). Left ventricular (LV) function was normal with an ejection fraction (EF) of 62%.

PCI procedure

Arterial access was obtained via the right femoral artery and 7500 IU heparin was administered. Through a 6 French (Fr) Cordis XB 3.5 guiding catheter, a 0.014 inch balance guidewire was passed across the lesion, which was predilated with a 2.5 × 15 mm Omnipass balloon to a maximum of

279

10 atmospheres, on two occasions sliding distally off the lesion. The guidewire was inadvertently pulled back and, although it remained across the lesion, it became apparent that there was a dissection that had propagated to beyond the wire tip. On attempting to advance the wire, the dissection extended more distally to involve a long segment of obtuse marginal artery (Fig. 50.2). With some difficulty, a 0.014 inch high-torque floppy wire was passed across the dissection and the proximal lesion redilated. However, as the dissection was long and the distal vessel small, we elected not to proceed further and to recall the patient for a follow-up angiography 1 month later. During the procedure the patient experienced some chest discomfort, but this had abated before she left the catheterization laboratory. Electrocardiography the following morning showed new T-wave inversion in leads I, III, AVF and V4-V6, and serum creatine kinase (CK) rose to 236 IU with a CK myocardial band (MB) of 21 IU, consistent with a non-Q-wave myocardial infarction. Over the following month she remained troubled by angina.

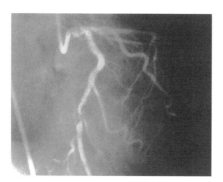

Figure 50.1. Lesion in the LCx artery prior to intervention.

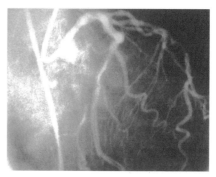

Figure 50.2. Long spiral dissection of the Cx artery extending distally.

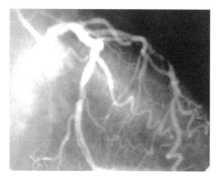

Figure 50.3. Appearance of the Cx artery at follow-up angiography 1 month after intervention.

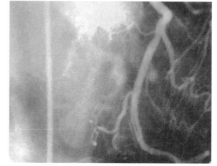

Figure 50.4. Successful stenting of the original proximal lesion.

The patient's readmission ECG showed resolution of the T-wave inversion. The follow-up angiogram revealed a patent artery with satisfactory flow but with a significant stenosis at the site of the original lesion (Fig. 50.3). This was successfully stented with a 3.0 × 16 mm NIR Primo stent without predilatation (Fig. 50.4). Her cardiac enzymes remained normal and she was discharged home the following morning.

Four months after the repeat procedure she remained asymptomatic.

Discussion

This case highlights the consequences of pulling back a coronary guidewire and the ease with which spiral dissections can occur. We also illustrate the ability of coronary dissections to 'heal' or 'tack-up' – a phenomenon that was often observed in the pre-stent era but is now seldom seen. We believe that in the situation of a long dissection extending into small diameter distal vessel, a conservative (non-stenting) approach should be considered, along with a repeat angiogram at a later time, with stenting of any residual stenosis. The time to the follow-up angiography should be long enough to allow the dissection to 'heal' but be balanced against the patient's symptomatic status.

Case 51

Rescue Angioplasty For Cardiogenic Shock Complicating Acute Myocardial Infarction (AMI): Extensive Vessel Thrombus Treated With Selective Injection Of Abciximab

Rodney H Stables

Background

A 43-year-old male was admitted to his local hospital with a sudden onset of severe central chest pain. The patient had no cardiac or other medical history of note and was taking no regular medications. Admission electrocardiograms (ECG) showed evidence of ST-segment elevation in the inferior leads and a diagnosis of AMI was made. Treatment was initiated with the administration of opiate analgesia, aspirin and thrombolysis with streptokinase.

Symptoms of chest pain persisted and repeat ECG suggested failure to reperfuse with no resolution of ST-segment abnormalities. Initial ST-segment depression in leads V1–V4 had been ascribed to so-called reciprocal change. Later tracings showed persistent ST-segment depression but also the development of new posterior Q-waves, manifest as initial R-wave deflections in the anterior leads. The infarct territory was therefore considered to be inferoposterior. Repeat thrombolysis with TPA was undertaken and the patient was transferred to the regional centre for further management.

Initial assessment after transfer suggested that repeat thrombolysis had not resulted in any improvement in the patient's pain or ECG abnormalities. Furthermore, there was evidence of acute left ventricular (LV) failure with systemic hypotension and clinical evidence of pulmonary oedema. He was transferred to the cardiac catheterization laboratory for further investigation and management.

On arrival in the catheterization laboratory, the patient was in low-output cardiogenic shock with frank LV failure. A pulmonary capillary-wedge pressure catheter was sited from the right femoral vein and confirmed elevation of the left atrial pressure with values of *c*. 25–30 mmHg. The systemic pressure, measured in the ascending aorta, was 70 mmHg. Diuretics were administered and an intraaortic balloon pump (IABP) sited via the left femoral artery.

Coronary arteriography revealed that the left main stem (LMS) was normal, the left anterior descending (LAD) coronary artery showed evidence of minor plaque disease but no focal stenoses. The circumflex (Cx) artery consisted of a single, large obtuse marginal branch (OMB). This was occluded proximally with evidence of thrombus propagation throughout the length of the vessel (Fig. 51.1).

The right coronary artery (RCA) was a dominant vessel, which exhibited diffuse disease throughout its course with two focal lesions. The more distal of these was just before the principal bifurcation. The other lesion was in the mid-vessel segment and was a tight stenosis with a ragged angiographic appearance, possibly representing the site of a recent occlusion, recanalized by thrombolytic therapy (Fig. 51.2). Despite these findings, normal TIMI grade 3 flow was present and initial angioplasty attempts were directed to the occluded Cx system.

A floppy guidewire (Cordis ATW) traversed the occluded segment in the Cx artery with ease. Initial balloon inflations were performed with an over-

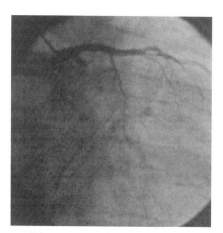

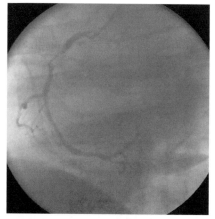

Figure 51.1. Left coronary system seen in posterio-anterior projection. The Cx vessel is occluded in its proximal portion.

Figure 51.2. Right coronary injection seen in the left anterior oblique (LAO) projection. A stenosis is seen in the distal vessel before the bifurcation, with more severe disease in the proximal part of the vertical segment.

the-wire angioplasty balloon (ACS Photon) matched to the vessel size. This had no appreciable impact on vessel patency or thrombus burden. Test injections of radiographic contrast through the guide catheter confirmed that introduction of abciximab by this route would have resulted in run-off of the drug down the patent LAD with no distribution to the Cx territory.

To counter this problem, an over-the-wire angioplasty balloon was advanced to the middle of the thrombosed portion of the vessel and intracoronary abciximab (ReoPro, Lilly) was administered. A slow hand-infusion of abciximab (standard, weight-adjusted bolus loading dose) was then introduced through the over-the-wire balloon, directly into the affected segment (Fig. 51.3). After 2–3 minutes this resulted in some restoration of coronary flow (TIMI grade 2 flow) and an improvement in the haemodynamic state (Fig. 51.4). Following delivery of the full bolus to the Cx coronary artery, abciximab was continued as an IV infusion.

Coronary angioplasty and stenting of the culprit lesions was then undertaken. The Cx coronary artery was treated with direct stent implantation using a 3.0 × 28 mm ACS Tetra stent at the previous occlusion site. An excellent angiographic result was obtained (Fig. 51.5).

In the RCA, the more distal stenosis (immediately before the bifurcation) was treated with the direct implantation of an ACS Tetra 3.0 × 23 mm stent. Then the occlusion site was treated with direct implantation of an ACS Tetra 4.0 × 28 mm stent. An excellent angiographic result was obtained.

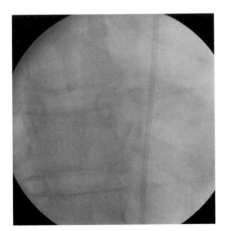 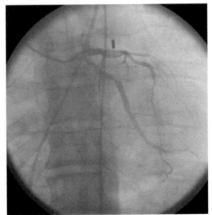

Figure 51.3. The over-the-wire angioplasty balloon is positioned in the occluded segment and the drug agent is injected through the central lumen into the affected region.

Figure 51.4. Following drug administration, anterograde flow is restored.

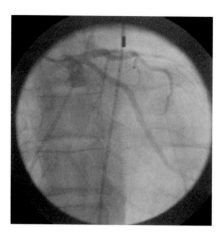

Figure 51.5. Final result following stent implantation.

No additional heparin was administered and all arterial lines and the IABP were removed 4 hours after the procedure. Haemostatsis was secured with manual pressure. The patient was initiated on routine secondary prevention medication. He mobilized on the ward without further evidence of heart failure or chest pain and was allowed home 6 days after admission.

Commentary

This case illustrates the potent therapeutic potential of abciximab in this setting. Selective delivery was achieved with application of over-the-wire balloon technology. I favour this type of balloon in the recanalization of occluded vessels. Over-the-wire balloons provide optimum wire support and the capability to exchange guidewires without losing position in the diseased segment. If the operator suspects that the passage of the guidewire may have created a dissection flap, the over-the-wire balloon can be advanced to a distal position. After removal of the guidewire, a radiographic contrast injection can be made through the central lumen of the balloon, which should delineate the true lumen of the distal vessel. Any wall staining confirms that the guidewire is in an abnormal plane. Interventionists and their trainees should remain familiar with the use of this type of balloon.

Case 52

CARDIOGENIC SHOCK DUE TO ACUTE LEFT MAIN OCCLUSION

Felix Zijlstra

Background

A 46-year-old male patient presented to the emergency room of a hospital, without invasive facilities, in profound cardiogenic shock with a systolic blood pressure of 72 mmHg and a heart rate of 114 beats/minute. He had developed sudden severe chest pain and dyspnea 1 hour before presentation. His electrocardiogram showed a sinus rhythm, right bundle branch block with left axis deviation, and ST elevation in all anterior and lateral leads. The patient was referred to and transported 30 km to our hospital.

Angiographic commentary

On arrival, the patient was brought directly to the catheterization laboratory, where he arrived *c.* 2 hours after symptom onset.

Coronary angiography showed a normal right coronary artery (RCA) (not shown) and a total occlusion of the left main coronary artery (LMCA) (Fig. 52.1). After balloon angioplasty and stenting (Fig. 52.2), patency of the artery was restored (Fig. 52.3). The patient was supported for 3 days with an intraaortic balloon pump. He made a full recovery and >1 year after the acute event he was asymptomatic and had resumed his former activities, except for smoking.

Discussion

Cardiogenic shock is a state of inadequate tissue perfusion due to cardiac dysfunction, most commonly caused by myocardial infarction.[1,2] Mortality rates for patients with cardiogenic shock remain very high, ranging from 50

287

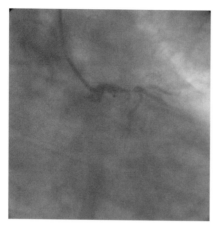

Figure 52.1. *27 September 2000, 13:13:19. Occlusion of LMCA with TIMI 1 flow.*

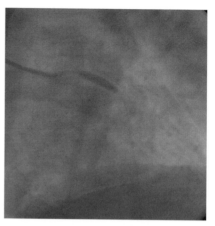

Figure 52.2. *27 September 2000, 13:15:19. Balloon inflation in the LMCA.*

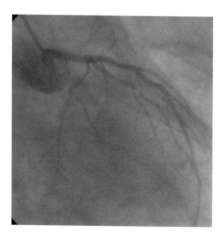

Figure 52.3. *27 September 2000, 13:16:55. Restoration of antegrade flow after balloon angioplasty and stenting.*

to 80%.[1,2] Recent estimates of the incidence of cardiogenic shock after myocardial infarction have ranged from 5 to 15%,[3] but the precise incidence is difficult to measure as many patients die before a diagnosis can be established.[1,3] A variety of causes may be involved, but pump failure due to a large infarction is the most common pathophysiological mechanism. Observational and randomized data show that early revascularization by angioplasty, in combination with hemodynamic support with an intraaortic balloon pump, improves early and long-term outcomes.[1,4]

In the SHOCK trial registry, the LMCA was the culprit vessel in 5.6% of patients and the associated mortality was 78.6%.[3] In the ULTIMA experience of angioplasty for left main occlusion during acute myocardial infarction

288

(AMI), 37 of 40 patients (92%) presented in cardiogenic shock, and in-hospital mortality was 55%.[5] Clinical outcome seemed to improve when stenting was performed after angioplasty.

Between 1990 and 1999, 20 patients with an acute occlusion of the LMCA were treated in the Isala Klinieken, Zwolle. Presentation was invariably cardiogenic shock. At 30 days, eight of 20 patients (40%) were alive, and survivors of the acute event recovered remarkably well. Ages of <60 years and treatment within 3 hours after symptom onset were predictive of survival. Three patients underwent elective bypass surgery for extensive triple-vessel disease and one patient underwent a second angioplasty procedure of the LMCA for restenosis, all within 4 months after the acute event.[6] Five patients remained asymptomatic during long-term follow-up without further interventions.

Cardiogenic shock due to acute total occlusion of the LMCA remains a challenge to the interventional cardiologist, but early and aggressive management can be life saving.

References

1. Hollenberg SM, Kavinsky CJ, Parrillo JE. Cardiogenic shock. *Ann Intern Med* 1999; **131**:47–59.

2. Hochman JS, Buller CE, Sleeper LA et al, for the SHOCK investigators. Cardiogenic shock complicating acute myocardial infarction – etiologies, management and outcome: a report from the SHOCK trial registry. *J Am Coll Cardiol* 2000; **36**:1063–70.

3. Wong SC, Sanborn T, Sleeper LA et al, for the SHOCK investigators. Angiographic findings and clinical correlates in patients with cardiogenic shock complicating acute myocardial infarction: a report from the SHOCK trial registry. *J Am Coll Cardiol* 2000; **36**:1077–83.

4. Sanborn TA, Sleeper LA, Bates ER et al, for the SHOCK investigators. Impact of thrombolysis, intraaortic balloon pump counterpulsation, and their combination in cardiogenic shock complicating acute myocardial infarction: a report from the SHOCK trial registry. *J Am Coll Cardiol* 2000; **36**:1123–9.

5. Marso SP, Steg G, Plokker T et al. Catheter-based reperfusion of unprotected left main stenosis during an acute myocardial infarction (the ULTIMATE experience). *Am J Cardiol* 1999; **83**:1513–17.

6. Stone GW, Brodie BR, Griffin JJ et al, for the primary angioplasty in myocardial infarction trial-2 (PAMI-2) investigators. Role of cardiac surgery in the hospital phase management of patients treated with primary angioplasty for acute myocardial infarction. *Am J Cardiol* 2000; **85**:1292–6.

289

Case 53

First Palmaz-Schatz Stent Implanted in Humans: 13-Year Angiography And Intravascular Ultrasound (IVUS) Follow-Up

J Eduardo Sousa, Alexandre Abizaid, Amanda GMR Sousa, Andrea Abizaid, Fausto Feres, Ibraim Pinto, Manoel Cano, Luiz Alberto Mattos, Luiz Fernando Tanajura, Julio Palmaz and Richard Schatz

Clinical history

This 56-year-old male, with history of dislipidemia and smoking presented in December 1987 with stable angina pectoris. Coronary angiography was performed and revealed a total occlusion in the mid portion of the right coronary artery (RCA) (Fig. 53.1). There was flow to the distal portion of the RCA from collaterals arising from the left system, which itself showed no significant lesions. The implantation of a new device, the Palmaz–Schatz stent, was selected as the revascularization strategy. After wire recanalization and balloon predilatation, the stent (hand-crimped) was deployed. The predilatation pressure was 6 atmospheres and the stent was deployed at 8 atmospheres. Post-stenting balloon dilatation was not performed. The final angiography image is shown in Fig. 53.2. The patient was discharged without complications 1 week after the index procedure; the antithrombotic regimen included aspirin 325 mg daily and dipiridamole 75 mg daily.

At 6 months, the patient underwent clinical and angiographic follow-up. He was asymptomatic and had a negative stress test. A minimal late loss was documented by coronary angiography (Fig. 53.3). Since then he has been followed annually with non-invasive tests, without evidence of ischemia.

In October 2000, the patient underwent angiographic and IVUS examinations, as shown in Figs 53.4 and 53.5. No significant disease had developed in the left system.

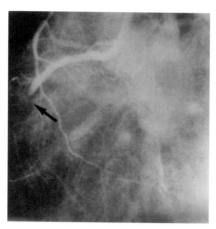

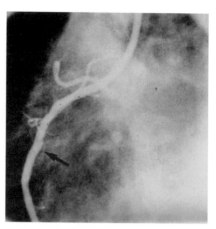

Figure 53.1. *Pre-procedure angiography, showing occlusion of the mid portion of the RCA.*

Figure 53.2. *Post-procedure angiography, showing a good angiographic result, with residual stenosis of 22%.*

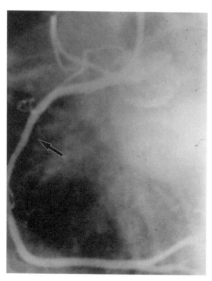

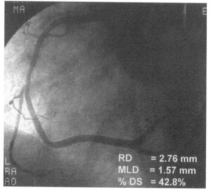

Figure 53.4. *Angiographic evaluation at 13 years, showing maintenance of the result at the dilated site. RD, Vessel reference diameter; MLD, minimal lumen diameter; %DS, percentage of stenosis.*

Figure 53.3. *Six months angiographic follow-up, showing maintenance of the result.*

Discussion

The significance of this case relies on the fact that this patient was the first human to be treated with an intracoronary Palmaz–Schatz stent. To our

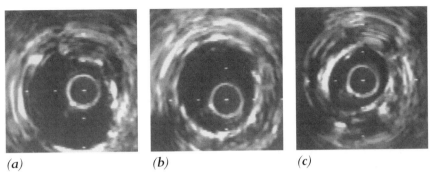

(a) *(b)* *(c)*

Figure 53.5. *(a) IVUS evaluation at the 13-year follow-up. The distal stent had a CSA of 8.81 mm^2, while the minimal lumen CSA was 8.17 mm^2. (b) The minimal lumen CSA was at the mid portion of the stent and measured 4.7 mm^2. The stent, which was clearly underexpanded, had a CSA at this site of 4.9 mm^2. (c) The proximal stent had a CSA of 9.23 mm^2, while the minimal lumen CSA was also 9.23 mm^2. The CSA of the mid portion of the stent (lesion site) was 45% less expanded than the proximal and distal ends of the prosthesis.*

knowledge, this is also the longest IVUS and angiographic follow-up of a patient with a coronary stent. Two points are relevant to this discussion:

- Because there was no previous experience with the use of stents, the final dilatation pressure was chosen on the basis of a good visual final result; this is the reason why the stent was deployed at a low pressure by current standards. The result of this strategy was evaluated at the 13-year follow-up when the first IVUS assessment was undertaken. The in-stent minimal cross-sectional area (CSA) was 4.9 mm^2, while the mean proximal and distal CSA was 9.02 mm^2 (Fig. 53.5). Remarkably, though, there was almost no intimal hyperplasia, suggesting that there was minimal neointimal proliferation in the 13 years of evolution. This finding may support the hypothesis that there is a direct relationship between the vessel wall injury and response, as proposed by Schwartz.[1,2]

- Also of relevance is the potential late effect of a metal prosthesis in the coronary arteries. In the early days of stent implantation, there were concerns as to whether the metal could oxidize and if a foreign-body reaction to the stent could develop. Even though the mid-term safety was confirmed at the 1-year follow-up angiographic studies,[3–5] the 13-year follow-up IVUS study was pivotal to document the absence of long-term negative reactions to the stent.

Therefore, this case gives a strong argument for a more widespread use of coronary stents, for they seem to maintain their good results over the long term, as documented here.

References

1. Schwartz RS. Pathophysiology of restenosis: interaction of thrombosis, hyperplasia, and/or remodeling. *Am J Cardiol* 1998; **81**:14E–17E.

2. Schwartz RS. The vessel wall reaction in restenosis. *Semin Intervent Cardiol* 1997; **2**:83–8.

3. Kimura T, Nosaka H, Yokoi H et al. Serial angiographic follow-up after Palmaz–Schatz stent implantation: comparison with conventional balloon angioplasty. *J Am Coll Cardiol* 1993; **21**:1557–63.

4. Kimura T, Yokoi H, Nakagawa Y et al. Three-year follow-up after implantation of metallic coronary-artery stents. *N Engl J Med* 1996; **334**:561–6.

5. Macaya C, Serruys PW, Ruygrok P et al. Continued benefit of coronary stenting versus balloon angioplasty: one-year clinical follow-up of Benestent trial. Benestent Study Group. *J Am Coll Cardiol* 1996; **27**:255–61.

Case 54

Intravascular Ultrasound (IVUS)-Guided Treatment Of In-Stent Restenosis: When Should The Interventionalist Consider Vessel Size Rather Than Lumen Size Alone?

Paul Schoenhagen, Patrick L Whitlow, Steven E Nissen and E Murat Tuzcu

Background

A 53-year-old male was referred for treatment of in-stent restenosis. Six months earlier a subtotal occlusion of the right coronary artery (RCA) had been reopened by rotablation and multiple stents (Fig. 54.1). The patient now presented with recurrent angina pectoris. Angiography showed diffuse in-stent restenosis (Fig. 54.2).

Angiographic commentary

The angiogram in Fig. 54.2 shows diffuse in-stent restenosis. A representative IVUS image (Fig. 54.3) shows the severity of neointimal proliferation, and also the stent and external elastic membrane (EEM) area. It is clear that the narrow lumen is not solely due to neointimal proliferation but also to underexpansion of the stent. The maximum increase in luminal size can therefore be achieved by removal of neointima and further stent expansion. The following images will exemplify an IVUS-guided approach to treatment (Figs 54.4–54.9).

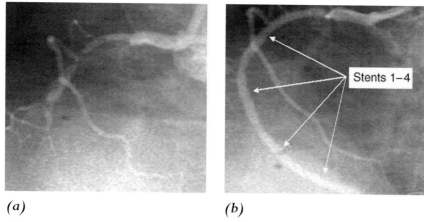

(a) *(b)*

Figure 54.1. *(a) The pre-interventional angiogram shows a subtotal occlusion of the RCA. Rotablation (1.25 mm burr) was complicated by a long dissection, which was treated with the deployment of four stents (3.0 × 18 mm; J&J stent). (b) The final angiogram demonstrates an excellent angiographic result. The diameter of the stented segment and the proximal reference measured 3 mm.*

Figure 54.2. Six months after this procedure described in Fig. 54.1, the patient returned with symptomatic diffuse in-stent restenosis, involving the entire stented segment. The angiographic lumen size of the mid-RCA measured 1.7 mm. The proximal reference size was 3.0 mm by angiography.

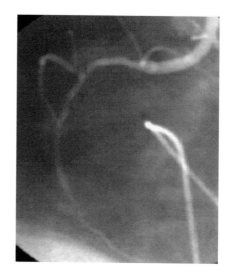

Discussion

In-stent restenosis is a very difficult clinical problem for which several different treatments have been proposed.[1-4] The presented case demonstrates a high-risk situation for restenosis because of the lesion length and diffuse disease. The success of treatment depends foremost on the lumen size

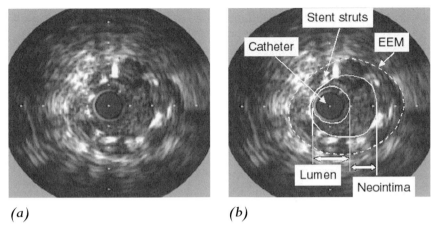

(a)   *(b)*

Figure 54.3. *(a) IVUS was performed. (b) The same image as in (a) but lumen, neointima, stent and EEM are labeled. Subsequently, rotablation was performed.*

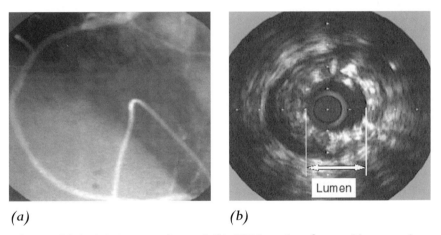

(a)   *(b)*

Figure 54.4. *(a) Angiographic and (b) IVUS results after rotablation with a 1.75 and 2.25 burr. The IVUS image after rotablation shows that the increased lumen size is achieved by reduction of neointimal volume.*

achieved at the end of the procedure and therefore every effort should be made to reach an optimally enlarged stent lumen.

True in-stent restenosis is caused mainly by neointimal growth,[5] however, the operator has to consider the possibility of stent underexpansion during the initial procedure. Therefore, treatment strategies can include removal of neointima and further stent expansion.[6,7]

297

Typically, the operator uses an angiographic reference site to decide about appropriate stent size and expansion. It is important to understand the rationale behind this approach. In a 'normal' reference, with minimal disease, lumen size is approximately equal to vessel size: therefore, reference lumen size is used to estimate lesion vessel size. IVUS studies have clearly documented the limitations of this approach. Several studies have demonstrated that reference sites often have significant disease.[8] The IVUS image of the 'reference' segment just proximal to the stent (Fig. 54.6) is a good example. It demonstrates a large plaque burden in a large-sized vessel. The small lumen size, which represents the angiographic reference size, significantly underestimates the vessel size. Based on this angiographic reference, stent dilatation would not have been considered.

The relationship between lumen and vessel size is further complicated because plaque progression and regression can lead to characteristic changes

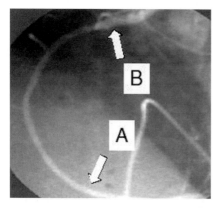

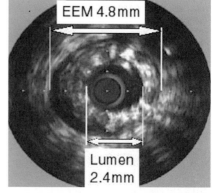

A

Figure 54.5. Angiogram and IVUS images of the lesion site and the proximal reference site after rotablation. The angiographic lumen size was 3 mm at the reference site (B) and 2.4 mm in the distal RCA (A), equivalent to an angiographic residual stenosis of 20%. However, the IVUS image demonstrates that the stent is underexpanded (in-stent lumen size 2.4 mm; EEM diameter 4.8 mm).

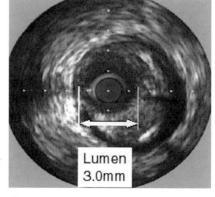

B

298

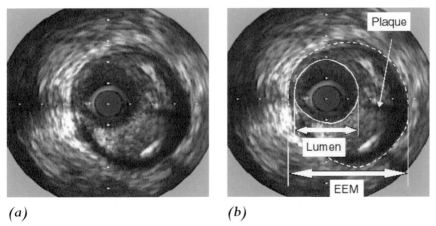

(a)   *(b)*

Figure 54.6. *IVUS image of the proximal reference segment (**a**) without and (**b**) with measurements. Because of a large plaque burden, the lumen size (3.0 mm) greatly underestimates vessel size (EEM 5.2 mm). The percentage area stenosis at the reference is 50%. [% area stenosis = (EEM$_{area}$ − lumen$_{area}$)/EEM$_{area}$ = 50]. Because of diffuse disease with involvement of the proximal reference, the comparison of angiographic lumen size at the lesion and reference site does not reveal stent underexpansion.*

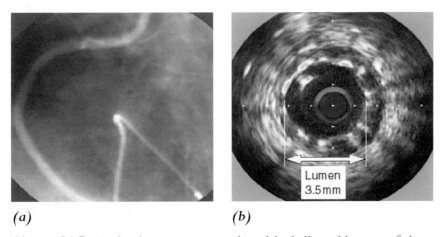

(a)   *(b)*

Figure 54.7. *Further lumen gain was achieved by balloon dilatation of the stent (3.5 × 40 mm Track Star balloon at 14 atmospheres). Angiographic and IVUS results after percutaneous transluminal coronary angioplasty (PTCA) are shown in (**a**) and (**b**), respectively.*

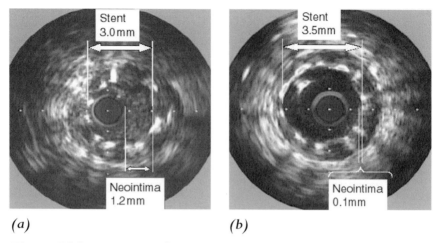

Figure 54.8. *Comparison of the IVUS images before (a) and after (b) intervention, showing the contribution of neointima reduction and stent dilatation to lumen gain.*

Figure 54.9. *A surveillance coronary angiogram 6 months later showed mild to moderate in-stent narrowing. The patient was asymptomatic.*

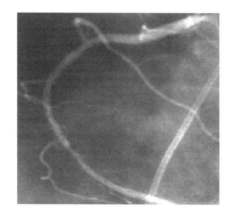

in vessel size, termed arterial remodeling. Plaque growth in early coronary artery disease is accommodated by vessel expansion rather than by lumen obstruction.[9] Arterial remodeling is clearly related to the clinical significance of atherosclerotic coronary lesions[10] and also influences the outcome of interventional procedures.[11,12]

Diffuse disease and remodeling are two major limitations of using the angiographic lumen size of the reference to estimate lesion vessel size. True vessel size can only be detected by IVUS, and recent studies show that this information can be used safely and effectively.[13–15] This case is an example of how knowledge of true vessel size can influence the interventional treatment strategy.

300

In summary, the interventionalist should always consider vessel size rather than lumen size alone.[16] In selected cases, the utilization of IVUS is helpful to guide therapy and achieve an optimal result.

References

1. Hoffmann R, Mintz GS, Dussaillant GR et al. Patterns and mechanisms of in-stent restenosis. *Circulation* 1996; **94**:1247–54.

2. Topaz O, Vetrovec GW. The stenotic stent: mechanisms and revascularization options. *Cathet Cardiovasc Diagn* 1996; **37**:293–9.

3. Stone GW. Rotational atherectomy for treatment of in-stent restenosis: role of intracoronary ultrasound guidance. *Cathet Cardiovasc Diagn* 1996; **3**:73–7.

4. Raizner AE, Oesterle SN, Waksman R et al. Inhibition of restenosis with beta-emitting radiotherapy. *Circulation* 2000; **102**:951–8.

5. Painter JA, Mintz GS, Wong SC et al. Serial intravascular ultrasound studies fail to show evidence of chronic Palmaz–Schantz stent recoil. *Am J Cardiol* 1995; **75**:398–400.

6. Kuntz RE, Gibson CM, Nobuyoshi M, Baim DS. Generalized model of restenosis after conventional balloon angioplasty, stenting and directional atherectomy. *J Am Coll Cardiol* 1993; **21**:15–25.

7. Beatt KJ, Serruys PW, Luijten HE et al. Restenosis after coronary angioplasty: the paradox of increased lumen diameter and restenosis. *J Am Coll Cardiol* 1992; **19**:258–66.

8. Mintz GS, Paanter JA, Pichard AL et al. Atherosclerosis in angiographically 'normal' coronary artery reference segments: an intravascular ultrasound study with clinical correlation. *J Am Coll Cardiol* 1995; **25**:1479–85.

9. Glagov S, Weisenberg E, Zarins CK et al. Compensatory enlargement of human atherosclerotic coronary arteries. *N Engl J Med* 1987; **316**:1371–53.

10. Schoenhagen P, Ziada KM, Kapadia SR et al. Extent and direction of arterial remodeling in stable and unstable coronary syndromes. *Circulation* 2000; **101**:598–603.

11. Dangas G, Mintz GS, Mehran R et al. Preintervention arterial remodeling as an independent predictor of target-lesion revascularization after nonstent coronary intervention. *Circulation* 1999; **99**:3149–54.

12. Dangas G, Mintz GS, Mehran R et al. Stent implantation neutralizes the impact of preintervention arterial remodeling on subsequent target lesion revascularization. *Am J Cardiol* 2000; **86**:452–5.

13. Stone GW, Hodgson JM, St Goar FG et al. Improved procedural results of coronary angioplasty with intravascular ultrasound-guided balloon sizing. The CLOUT pilot trial. *Circulation* 1997; **95**:2044–52.

14. Fitzgerald PJ, Oshima A, Hayase M et al. Final results of the routine ultrasound can influence stent expansion (CRUISE) study. *Circulation* 2000; **102**:523–30.

15. Frey AW, Hodgson JM, Mueller C et al. Ultrasound-guided strategy for provisional stenting with focal balloon combination catheter. *Circulation* 2000; **102**:2497–502.

16. Topol EJ, Nissen SE. Our preoccupation with coronary luminology. *Circulation* 1995; **92**:2333–42.

Case 55

QUESTIONS AND ANSWERS – 1: UNSTABLE ANGINA AND MULTIVESSEL DISEASE (MVD) – 1

Morton Kern

A 58-year-old physician who had percutaneous transluminal coronary angioplasty (PTCA) and stenting in the right coronary artery (RCA) in 1998 had complained of resting angina for 3 days.

Question 1

What is the most appropriate first step in the evaluation of this patient with coronary artery disease who had a previous stent placed?

(a)   exercise electrocardiographic stress testing
(b)   increase statin drugs and observe
(c)   increase angiotensin-converting-enzyme (ACE) inhibitors and monitor blood pressure
(d)   perform cardiac catheterization
(e)   perform cardiac catheterization and give clopidogrel.

Answer: (e).

Patients with stents who have typical angina, especially resting angina, months after their procedure have a high likelihood of having in-stent restenosis or, alternatively, a new and severe atherosclerotic narrowing elsewhere.

(a)   Exercise testing is relatively contraindicated in resting angina.
(b)   and (c) Statins and ACE inhibitors must be optimized but one should not move from one to the other when making a diagnosis.

Coronary angiography is also recommended to be performed.

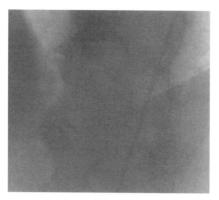

Figure 55.1. *Left anterior oblique (LAO) view of the LAD artery, showing intermediate narrowing of the mid-vessel segment.*

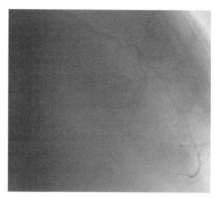

Figure 55.2. *Right anterior oblique (RAO) view of the LAD artery, showing intermediate narrowing of the mid-vessel segment.*

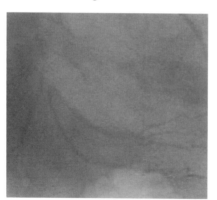

Figure 55.3. *RAO view showing a severe new lesion in the Cx artery.*

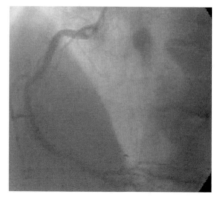

Figure 55.4. *LAO view of the RCA, showing new narrowing distal to the stent.*

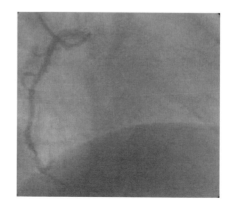

Figure 55.5. *LAO view of the RCA.*

304

Question 2

Which artery is the 'culprit' vessel responsible for angina?

(a)   right coronary artery (RCA)
(b)   left anterior descending (LAD)
(c)   circumflex (Cx)
(d)   cannot determine from angiograms.

Answer: (d).

Angiography is limited to determining if coronary blood flow is impaired.

Question 3

What is the next most appropriate step for this patient?

(a)   continue medical therapy and perform out-of-laboratory stress testing
(b)   angioplasty of all lesions
(c)   coronary artery bypass graft (CABG) surgery
(d)   visually select 'culprit' lesion by taking more angiographic views
(e)   physiologically assess lesion severity in catheterization laboratory to determine which are suitable for PTCA.

Answer: (e).

(a)   No stress testing is to be performed in unstable angina.
(b)   The LAD lesion does not look severe, no PTCA based on visual lesion severity.
(c)   Same approach as (b) for CABG.
(d)   More angiography would not be helpful.

Question 4

What method would be most suitable to assess lesion severity in the catheterization laboratory?

(a)   coronary flow velocity reserve (CFUR)
(b)   pressure-derived fractional flow reserve (FFR)
(c)   relative coronary flow reserve (rCFR)
(d)   intravascular ultrasound (IVUS)
(e)   QCA-derived TIMI frame count.

Answer: (b).

FFR is performed for all three vessels.

(a)   CFVR would be helpful only if normal, >2.0, but uncertainty about this value is large.

(b)   rCFR cannot be used since there is no normal reference artery to measure.

(d)   IVUS is not a physiologic measurement, only anatomic.

(e)   TIMI frame count is not physiologic for lesion assessment.

Question 5

FFR is 0.73, 0.68 and 0.64 for the LAD, Cx and RCA, respectively. Based on these data, what is the next most appropriate step?

(a)   continue medical therapy

(b)   angioplasty of all lesions

(c)   CABG

(d)   Angioplasty of only the RCA and Cx

(e)   Mid-CABG for LAD only.

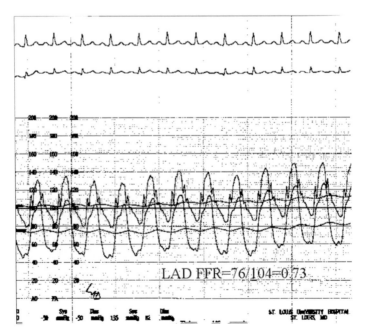

LAD FFR=76/104=0.73

Figure 55.6.

306

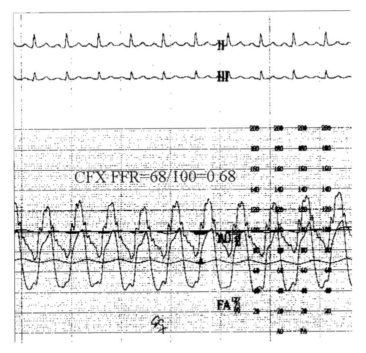

Figure 55.7.

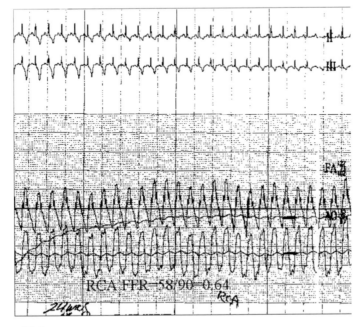

Figure 55.8.

Answer: (c).

(a) All FFR values <0.75 indicate significant association with inducible ischemia.

(b) PTCA of all lesions is difficult and unsatisfactory results are likely, especially for the Cx.

(d) The RCA and the Cx are significant ischemia-producing lesions too.

(e) The LAD also needs intervention based on FFR.

Case 56

Questions And Answers – 2: Unstable Angina And Multivessel Disease (MVD) – 2

Morton Kern

A 72-year-old male with end-stage renal disease who is on dialysis is being evaluated for a renal transplant. He is relatively asymptomatic without chest pain, paroxysmal nocturnal dysnea (PND), significant dysnea on exertion (DOE), dyspnea or pedal edema. He has no prior history of coronary artery disease.

Question 1

What is the appropriate evaluation for this patient?

(a) exercise electrocardiographic stress
(b) exercise stress echo
(c) dobutamine stress echo
(d) cardiac catheterization
(e) resting 2D and Doppler echo.

Answer: (b).

(a) In renal patients, hypertension is common and electrocardiograms (ECG) are not accurate for ischemic changes.
(c) Dobutamine echo is not as good as exercise stress echo but is an acceptable alternative.
(d) May be performed after stress echo if necessary. If stress test normal, a catheter is not needed in an asymptomatic patient.
(e) Resting echo is not helpful for ischemia.

No stress test was performed but the patient was sent directly to the cardiac catheterization laboratory. Coronary angiography was performed. Left ventriculography was normal. The right coronary artery (RCA) was also normal. The left coronary artery (LCA) images are shown.

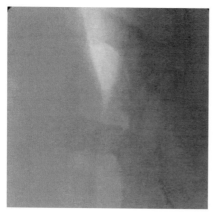

Figure 56.1. *Left anterior oblique (LAO) view of the LAD artery.*

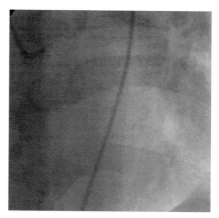

Figure 56.2. *Right anterior oblique (RAO) view of the LAD artery.*

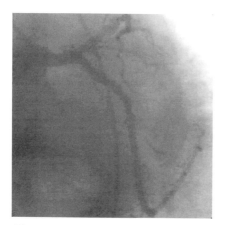

Figure 56.3. *LAO caudal view.*

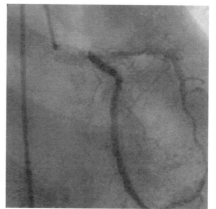

Figure 56.4. *RAO view of the LAD artery.*

Question 2

Based on the angiograms, which of the following statements is correct?
(a) the left main stenosis is critically narrowed
(b) the circumflex (Cx) artery is critically narrowed
(c) the left main stenosis is not severe
(d) the LAD is critically narrowed
(e) the left main is of an uncertain degree of obstruction.

Answer: (e).

The left main lesion is severe in one view and mild in the orthogonal view.

Question 3

What is the next most appropriate step in this patient?

(a) proceed to renal transplant
(b) coronary artery bypass graft (CABG) then renal transplant
(c) angioplasty of left main
(d) defer intervention, move from laboratory and do a stress test
(e) assess lesion in laboratory.

Answer: (e).

(a) Uncertainty of left main severity needs to be resolved before transplant.
(b) and (c) Should not be undertaken without more objective information than angiogram.
(d) An out-of-laboratory test wastes time and resources.

Question 4

What method would be most suitable to assess the left main lesion severity in the catheterization laboratory?

(a) coronary flow velocity reserve (CFVR)
(b) pressure-derived fractional flow reserve (FFR)
(c) relative coronary flow reserve (rCFR)
(d) intravascular ultrasound (IVUS)
(e) QCA-derived TIMI frame count

Answer: (b) or (d).

(a) CFVR would be helpful only if normal, >2.0, but uncertainty about this value is large.
(c) rCFR cannot be used since there is no normal reference artery to measure.
(d) IVUS is not a physiologic measurement only anatomic; however, cross-sectional areas (CSA) $<4.0\,mm^2$ are considered to be physiologically important.
(e) TIMI frame count is not physiological for lesion assessment.

311

Figure 56.5. *IVUS; FFR = 0.94.*

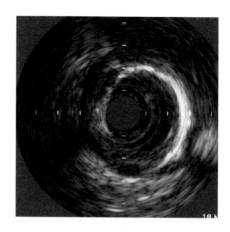

Question 5

Based on IVUS and FFR data, what is the next most appropriate step in this patient?

(a)   proceed to renal transplant
(b)   CABG then renal transplant
(c)   angioplasty of left main
(d)   defer intervention, move from laboratory and do a stress test
(e)   assess lesion in laboratory.

Answer: (a).

The IVUS showed large CSA ($>12\,mm^2$) and the FFR was completely normal (0.94). This eccentric calcified narrowing of the left main is not hemodynamically significant and would not benefit from revascularization at this time.

INDEX

Notes: Page numbers in *italics* refer to figures and/or tables. Abbreviations used in subentries are defined in main entries.

317

319